£34.99.

MR **S**

MRCPCH Part 2 Practice Exams
– Third edition

Dr Giles Kendall

MB BS BSc(Hons) MRCPCH
Research Fellow
Centre For Perinatal Brain Protection and Repair
University College London

Dr Ian Pollock

MBBS MRCP FRCPCH DCH DRCOG
Consultant Paediatrician
Chase Farm Hospital
Barnet and Chase Farm Hospitals NHS Trust
Enfield, Middlesex

© 2004 PasTest Ltd
Egerton Court
Parkgate Estate
Knutsford
Cheshire, WA16 8DX

Telephone: 01565 752000

First edition 1993
Second edition 1999
Third edition 2004

ISBN: 1 901198 871

A catalogue record for this book is available from the British Library.

The information contained within this book was obtained by the authors from
reliable sources. However, while every effort has been made to ensure its accuracy,
no responsibility for loss, damage or injury occasioned to any person acting or
refraining from action as a result of information contained herein can be accepted
by the publisher or the authors.

PasTest Revision Books and Intensive Courses
PasTest has been established in the field of postgraduate medical education since
1972, providing revision books and intensive study courses for doctors preparing
for their professional examinations. Books and courses are available for the
following specialties:

MRCP Part 1 and Part 2, MRCPCH Part 1 and Part 2, MRCOG, DRCOG, MRCGP,
MRCPsych, DCH, FRCA, MRCS and PLAB.

For further details contact:

PasTest Ltd, Freepost, Knutsford, Cheshire, WA16 7BR
Tel: 01565 752000   Fax: 01565 650264
Email: enquiries@pastest.co.uk   **Web site: www.pastest.co.uk**

Typeset by Saxon Graphics Ltd, Derby
Printed by Cambrian Printers, Aberystwyth

CONTENTS

AUTHORS OF FIRST AND SECOND EDITIONS

Dr Mike Greenberg
MRCP MRCPCH
Consultant Paediatrician
Royal Free Hospital
London

Dr P Gringras
Consultant Paediatrician
Multiple Births Foundation
Queen Charlotte's Hospital
London
Harper House Children's Service
Hertfordshire

Dr D K Pal
Specialist Registrar in Paediatric Neurology
Great Ormond Street Children's Hospital
London

INTRODUCTION

The new examination

In 1999 the recently formed Royal College of Paediatrics and Child Health established their own membership examination. Until July 2002 the format of the examination followed that of its predecessor, the MRCP (UK), with separate papers examining Case Histories, Data Interpretation, and Photographic Material.

In 2002 there was a change from three to two papers, each consisting of a mixture of question types and an extended curriculum to include research, audit, ethics, and medical science applied to clinical care. The style of questions was also changed to multiple choice, extended matching and 'n' from many, along with the introduction of a computerised mark sheet.

About this book

Questions have been set out in the form of five individual exams. They are a mixture of question types and have been extensively revised to take into account the changes in the exam format and curriculum. Many questions have been retained and adapted from previous editions as they cover topics that remain relevant to the examination. Picture tests and integrated questions have been added to make the papers as representative as possible. The explanations aim to provide frameworks for problem solving and pattern recognition. It is hoped that this book will be a valuable tool in the preparation for the challenge of the MRCPCH.

Giles Kendall

MRCPCH PART 2 EXAMINATION

Practice Exam 1

Answer all 15 questions in the allotted time (2½ hours). At the end of each question the value of that question is shown in brackets. The total mark for this paper is 48.

QUESTION 1.1

A 14-year-old girl is under paediatric follow-up following a referral 3 years ago for investigation of short stature. She was diagnosed as having anorexia nervosa 2 years ago, soon after her menarche. Since then, despite behavioural and family therapy she has remained anorexic and has been amenorrhoeic for the last year.

On examination she is thin, other than the oral features shown. The examination of the other systems is normal.

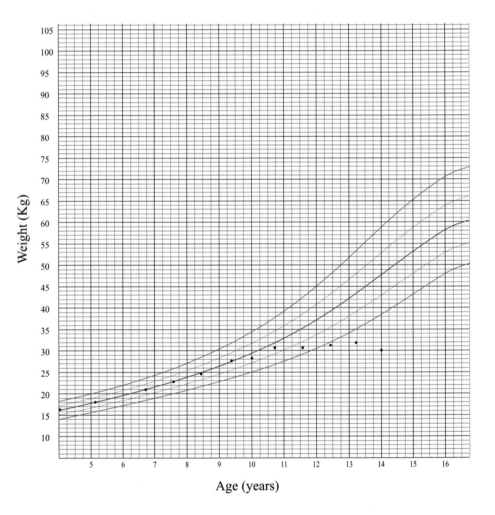

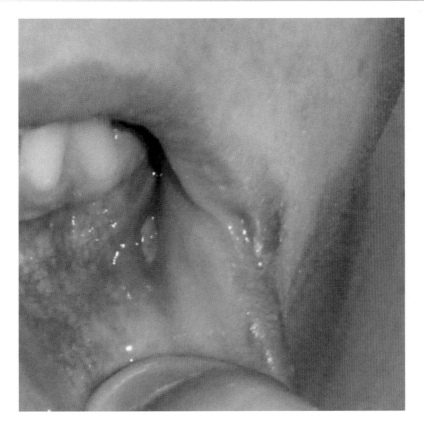

Investigations

Blood pressure normal
Urinalysis normal
Full blood count:

Hb	9.5 g/dl
WBC	12.1 × 10⁹/litre
Platelets	320 × 10⁹/litre
MCH	26 pg
MCVfL	76
ESR:	40 mm/hour
Sodium	136 mmol/litre
Potassium	3.6 mmol/litre
Urea	3.1 mmol/litre

a) What further investigation would be most useful in making a diagnosis? (maximum 2 marks)

Select ONE answer only

- ☐ A Barium meal and follow-through
- ☐ B T cell subsets
- ☐ C Anti-endomysial antibodies
- ☐ D Bone marrow aspiration
- ☐ E Pituitary function testing
- ☐ F Colonoscopy and biopsy

b) What is the most likely diagnosis? (1 mark)

Select ONE answer only

- ☐ A Coeliac disease
- ☐ B Pituitary insufficiency
- ☐ C Human immune deficiency virus
- ☐ D Crohn's disease
- ☐ E Anorexia nervosa

QUESTION 1.2

A baby was born prematurely at 31 weeks. He required one dose of surfactant and continuous positive airway pressure (CPAP) for 2 days; 12 hours after stopping CPAP and commencing feeds, he became tachypnoeic and appeared pale. Feeds were stopped for 6 hours and he settled with CPAP. At 4 days of age he becomes apnoeic requiring intubation and ventilation. Jerking movements are noted whilst the baby is on the ventilator.

Investigations

Blood glucose: 2.4 mmol/litre
Urea and electrolytes normal
Arterial blood gas:

pH   7.1
PaO_2 10 kPa
$PaCO_2$ 5.1 kPa
Base excess –17 mmol/litre

a) **What three investigations should be performed immediately?**
   (3 marks)

Select THREE answers only

- [ ] A Blood culture
- [ ] B Urine toxicology screen
- [ ] C Lumbar puncture for CSF glucose/protein/culture
- [ ] D Congenital viral screen
- [ ] E Cranial ultrasound scan
- [ ] F Amino and organic acids screen
- [ ] G C-reactive protein
- [ ] H Upper GI contrast study
- [ ] I Serum calcium and magnesium levels
- [ ] J Full blood count

Following investigation the child is commenced on intravenous antibiotics, a fluid bolus of 20 ml/kg of normal saline is given and, following some further jerking movements, a loading dose of phenobarbitone is given. Feeds are stopped and maintenance iv fluids are commenced.

b) **What is the most likely diagnosis? (1 mark)**

Select ONE answer only

☐ A Duodenal atresia
☐ B Sepsis and meningitis
☐ C Inborn error of metabolism
☐ D Neonatal narcotic withdrawal syndrome
☐ E Hypoxic ischaemic encephalopathy

QUESTION 1.3

A 14-year-old girl presents to A&E with generalised malaise, lethargy and a sore throat. On examination the following oral findings are present.

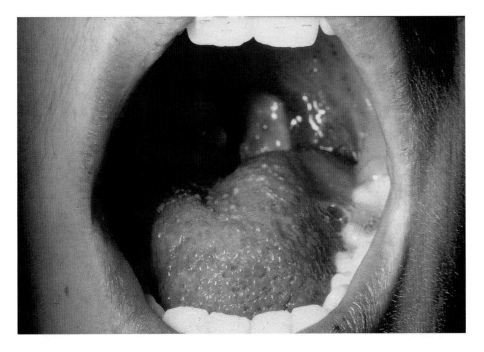

a) What diagnostic investigation would be of most value? (1 mark)

Select ONE answer only

- [ ] A Full blood count
- [ ] B Monospot test
- [ ] C Throat swab culture
- [ ] D Herpes simplex serology
- [ ] E Bone marrow aspirate

QUESTION 1.4

A 9-year-old boy presents with a 2-week history of unproductive cough and pain over the right chest wall. He has been treated for a chest infection with ampicillin for 1 week. The child is getting worse with a poor appetite, weight loss, headache and dizziness.

Father is a postman, mother had pneumonia responding to antibiotics 2 weeks ago. His 7-year-old brother is well and the family lives in a two-room council flat with a cat and a budgie.

On examination he is pyrexial at 40°C and looks ill. His pulse rate is 170 and his capillary refill time mildly prolonged. There is reduced chest expansion on the right side of the chest, with dullness to percussion, reduced breath sounds and crackles heard in the right lower zone.

A chest X-ray is obtained:

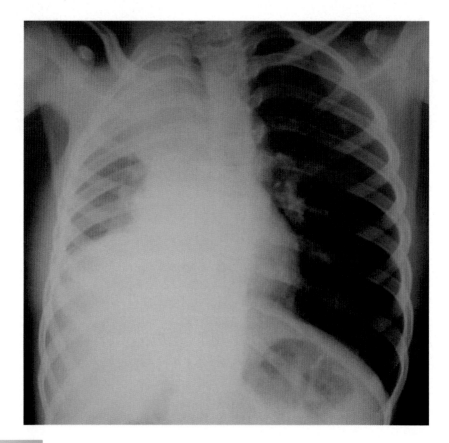

a) What best describes the X-ray appearance? (1 mark)

Select ONE answer only

- ☐ A Right lower lobe consolidation
- ☐ B Right lower lobe consolidation with collapse
- ☐ C Right upper lobe consolidation
- ☐ D Right upper lobe consolidation with collapse
- ☐ E Right pleural effusion
- ☐ F Right pleural effusion with upper lobe consolidation
- ☐ G Right pleural effusion with lower lobe consolidation

Other investigations are performed:
Hb: 8.5 g/dl
WBC: 6.2×10^9/litre
ESR: 65 mm/hour
Heaf test: grade I

b) What two diagnostic investigations would you perform next? (2 marks)

Select TWO answers only

- ☐ A Pleural tap for microscopy and culture of any fluid
- ☐ B Bronchoscopy and bronchoalveolar lavage
- ☐ C Early morning gastric washings for mycobacterium
- ☐ D Reticulocyte count
- ☐ E Specific serological testing
- ☐ F CT scan of the chest
- ☐ G Blood culture
- ☐ H Cold agglutinins
- ☐ I Mantoux test

c) What is the treatment of choice? (1 mark)

Select ONE answer only

- ☐ A   Combination antituberculous therapy
- ☐ B   Oral macrolide antibiotic
- ☐ C   Intravenous broad spectrum antibiotic, eg cefuroxime
- ☐ D   Intravenous flucloxacillin
- ☐ E   Intravenous co-trimoxazole

QUESTION 1.5

Consider the following list of research techniques.

A   Cross-sectional study
B   Geographical study
C   Cohort study
D   Case control study
E   Randomised control trial
F   Clinical audit
G   Outcome audit

a)   Choose the most appropriate study from the list above for the investigation of the following situations. (1 mark each, total 7 marks). Each answer may be used once, more than once or not at all.

Select ONE answer only for each situation

- [ ] 1. Evaluation of a new drug in comparison with an existing treatment
- [ ] 2. Calculation of prevalence
- [ ] 3. Evaluation of clinical practice
- [ ] 4. Estimation of incidence
- [ ] 5. Calculation of the relative risk of a disease related to risk factors
- [ ] 6. The study of cause in a rare disease
- [ ] 7. Establishing a temporal sequence

QUESTION 1.6

A child is brought to A&E with the rash shown below; 2 weeks ago he was seen for a sore throat and was treated with ibuprofen.

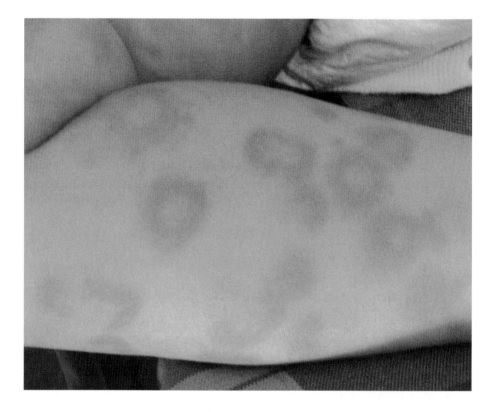

a) What is the most likely diagnosis? (1 mark)

Select ONE answer only

- ☐ A Erythema nodosum
- ☐ B Urticaria
- ☐ C Pityriasis rosea
- ☐ D Erythema multiforme
- ☐ E Herpes simplex

QUESTION 1.7

Examine this audiogram of a 2-year-old with delayed speech.

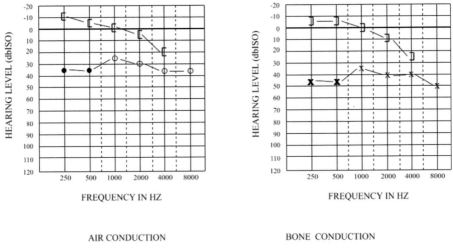

AIR CONDUCTION   BONE CONDUCTION

O RIGHT   X LEFT   [MASKED RIGHT   ] MASKED LEFT

● MASKED   ✗ MASKED

a) What abnormality is revealed? (1 mark)

Select ONE answer only

- ☐ A Left moderate conductive hearing loss
- ☐ B Left severe conductive hearing loss
- ☐ C Left severe sensorineural hearing loss
- ☐ D Right moderate conductive hearing loss
- ☐ E Right severe conductive hearing loss
- ☐ F Right severe sensorineural hearing loss
- ☐ G Bilateral moderate conductive hearing loss
- ☐ H Bilateral moderate sensorineural hearing loss
- ☐ I Bilateral severe conductive hearing loss
- ☐ J Bilateral severe sensorineural hearing loss

b) Suggest the most likely cause for this. (1 mark)

Select ONE answer only

- [ ] A Alport's syndrome
- [ ] B Hearing loss post meningitis
- [ ] C Acute otitis media
- [ ] D Chronic suppurative otitis media
- [ ] E Otosclerosis

QUESTION 1.8

Consider the following family tree.

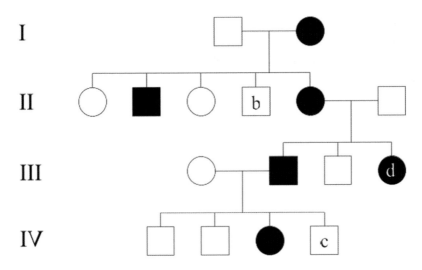

a) **What best describes the pattern of inheritance shown? (maximum 2 marks)**

Select ONE answer only

- [ ] A Autosomal dominant
- [ ] B Autosomal recessive
- [ ] C X-linked dominant
- [ ] D X-linked recessive
- [ ] E Mitochondrial

Consider the following list of probabilities.

A Zero
B < 1%
C 1%
D 5%
E 25%
F 50%
G 67%
H 100%

b) Choose the most appropriate risk from the list on p. 17 for the following situations. (1 mark each, total 4 marks). Each answer may be used once, more than once or not at all.

Select ONE answer only for each situation

☐ 1. What is the chance of individual *b* having the disease?

☐ 2. What is the chance of individual *c* having the disease?

☐ 3. What is the chance that male offspring of the individual *d* have the disease?

☐ 4. What is the chance that female offspring of the individual *d* have the disease?

QUESTION 1.9

An infant is brought to A&E with the rash shown below. He has been generally unwell for a few days but is now apyrexial and happy.

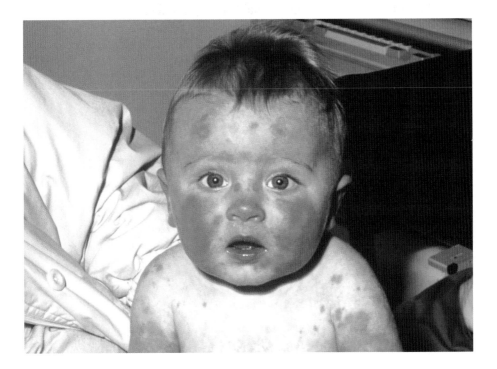

a) What is the most likely causative organism? (1 mark)

Select ONE answer only

☐ A Parvovirus B19
☐ B *Staphylococcus aureus*
☐ C Human herpes virus type 6
☐ D Rubella
☐ E *Borrelia burgdorferi*

QUESTION 1.10

A child being investigated for developmental delay and abnormal movements undergoes an EEG investigation.

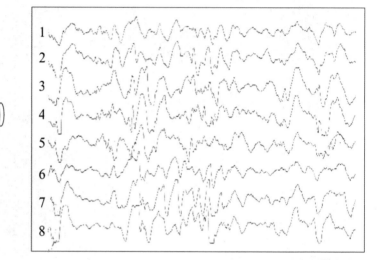

a) What pattern is shown? (1 mark)

Select ONE answer only

- ☐ A   3-per-second spike and wave activity
- ☐ B   Subacute sclerosing panencephalitis
- ☐ C   Generalised encephalopathy
- ☐ D   Hypsarrhythmia
- ☐ E   Benign rolandic epilepsy

A cranial CT scan is also performed:

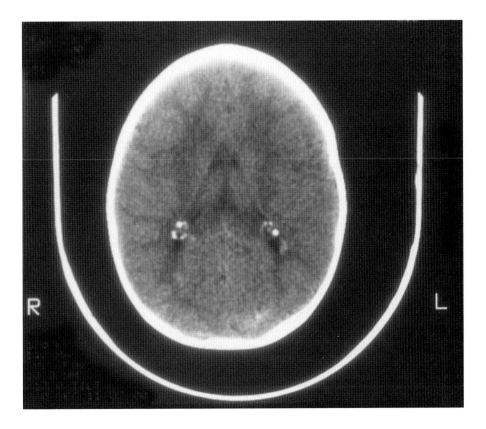

b) **What is the most likely diagnosis? (1 mark)**

Select ONE answer only

☐ A Subacute sclerosing panencephalitis
☐ B Sturge–Weber syndrome
☐ C Von Hippel–Lindau syndrome
☐ D Tuberous sclerosis
☐ E Congenital rubella

QUESTION 1.11

A 4-month-old girl presents with failure to thrive and poor feeding. The ECG taken is shown below.

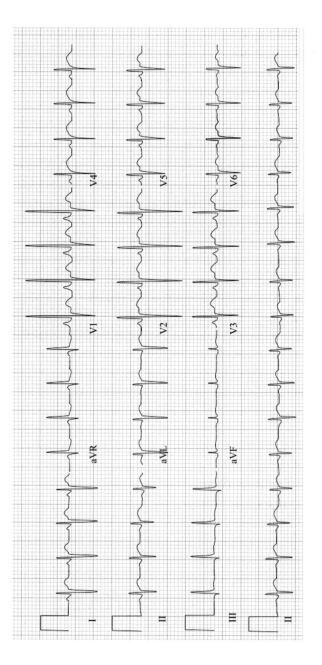

a) What three abnormalities are shown on the ECG? (3 marks)

Select THREE answers only

☐ A Right axis deviation
☐ B Left axis deviation
☐ C Right atrial enlargement
☐ D Left atrial enlargement
☐ E 1st degree heart block
☐ F 2nd degree heart block
☐ G Left ventricular hypertrophy
☐ H Right ventricular hypertrophy

The girl undergoes a cardiac catheter procedure:

Site	O₂ Saturation (%)	Pressure (mmHg)
S.V.C.	75	4
I.V.C.	74	
R.A.	75	
R.V.	90	90/8
P.A.	90	20/4
L.A.	90	6
L.V.	89	92/10

b) What two abnormalities are present? (2 marks)

Select TWO answers only

☐ A Atrial septal defect
☐ B Ventricular septal defect
☐ C Left ventricular hypertrophy
☐ D Right ventricular hypertrophy
☐ E Left ventricular outflow obstruction
☐ F Right ventricular outflow obstruction
☐ G Patent ductus arteriosus
☐ H Atrioventricular discordance

c) What is the most likely diagnosis? (1 mark)

Select ONE answer only

- [ ] A Transposition of the great arteries
- [ ] B Truncus arteriosus
- [ ] C Tetralogy of Fallot
- [ ] D Total anomalous pulmonary venous drainage
- [ ] E Ebstein's anomaly

d) What emergency procedure might a symptomatic infant suffering with this condition require? (1 mark)

Select ONE answer only

- [ ] A Balloon atrial septostomy
- [ ] B Blalock–Taussig shunt
- [ ] C Pulmonary artery banding
- [ ] D Closure of septal defect
- [ ] E Ligation of ductus arteriosus

QUESTION 1.12

A 13-year-old boy presents with a history of recurrent left-sided knee pain, worse when playing football and the appearance shown below.

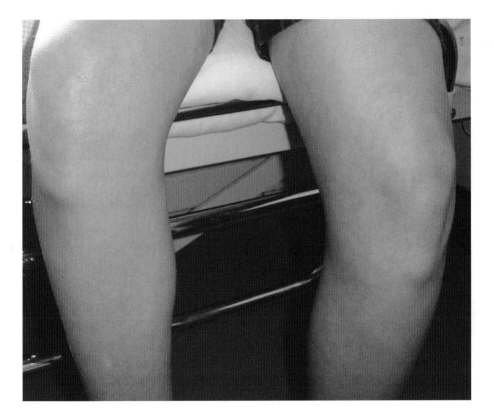

a) **What is the most likely diagnosis? (1 mark)**

Select ONE answer only

- [ ] A Proximal tibial osteomyelitis
- [ ] B Infrapatellar bursitis
- [ ] C Patellar tendonitis
- [ ] D Dislocated patella
- [ ] E Osgood–Schlatter disease

QUESTION 1.13

A 13-year-old boy from Ireland presents to A&E with tiredness and lethargy; he has been unwell for around 4 days with non-specific symptoms. On examination he appears pale and unwell. Observations include:

Temperature: 37.6°C
HR: 124
RR: 35
Sats: 98% in air
Chest clear
Heart sounds: ejection systolic murmur

The remainder of the examination is unremarkable. Other than an episode of jaundice 4 years ago he has remained well. His father has also had a number of recurrent episodes of jaundice.

Investigations

Hb:	4.0 g/dl
WBC:	5.4 × 10⁹/litre
Platelets:	120 × 10⁹/litre
Na:	136 mmol/litre
K:	3.8 mmol/litre

Following a blood transfusion he makes a complete recovery. Further investigations are arranged as an outpatient because of slight discoloration of the sclera.

Investigations

Total bilirubin:	60 μmol/litre
Conjugated bilirubin:	3 μmol/litre
Total protein:	66 g/litre
ALT:	13 IU/litre
ALP:	120 IU/litre
Haptoglobin:	0.1 g/litre (0.3–2 g/litre)
Hb:	9.0 g/dl
WBC:	8.4 × 10⁹/litre
Platelets:	325 × 10⁹/litre

a) What is this child's underlying diagnosis: (1 mark)

Select ONE answer only

- [ ] A Hereditary spherocytosis
- [ ] B Pyruvate kinase deficiency
- [ ] C Hereditary elliptocytosis
- [ ] D Glucose-6-phosphate dehydrogenase deficiency
- [ ] E Diamond–Blackfan syndrome

b) What one diagnostic investigation could confirm this? (1 mark)

Select ONE answer only

- [ ] A Red cell enzyme analysis
- [ ] B Bone marrow aspiration
- [ ] C Osmotic fragility testing
- [ ] D Blood film
- [ ] E Chromosome analysis

c) What was the most likely cause of his acute illness? (1 mark)

Select ONE answer only

- [ ] A Hepatitis A
- [ ] B Human herpes virus 6
- [ ] C Epstein–Barr virus
- [ ] D *Mycoplasma pneumoniae*
- [ ] E Parvovirus B19

QUESTION 1.14

Consider the following list of biochemical combinations.

	Calcium	Phosphate	ALP	Parathyroid	25 (OH) Vit D
A	Low	Low	Low	High	Normal
B	Low	Low/normal	High	High	Normal
C	Normal/low	High	High	High	Normal
D	High	High	High	Low	Low
E	High	Low	Normal/high	High	Normal
F	Low/normal	Low/normal	High	High	Low
G	Normal	Very Low	High	Normal	Normal/low

Choose the most appropriate combination from the list above for the following conditions. (1 mark each, total 5 marks). Each answer may be used once, more than once or not at all.

Select ONE answer only for each situation

- ☐ 1. Primary hyperparathyroidism
- ☐ 2. Secondary hyperparathyroidism
- ☐ 3. X-linked hypophosphataemic rickets
- ☐ 4. Vitamin D-deficient rickets
- ☐ 5. Vitamin D-dependent rickets

QUESTION 1.15

Consider this photograph of a teenage boy looking straight ahead.

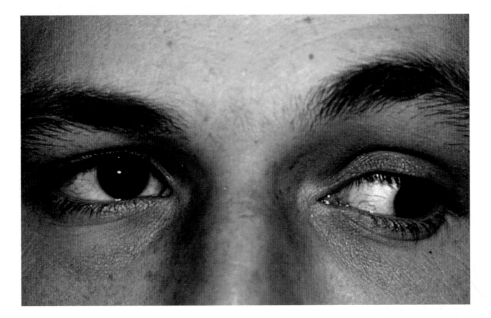

a) What is the diagnosis? (1 mark)

Select ONE answer only

- [ ] A Right convergent squint
- [ ] B Left 3rd cranial nerve palsy
- [ ] C Left 4th cranial nerve palsy
- [ ] D Left 6th cranial nerve palsy
- [ ] E Left Horner's syndrome

MRCPCH PART 2 EXAMINATION

Practice Exam 2

Answer all 15 questions in the allotted time (2½ hours). At the end of each question the value of that question is shown in brackets. The total mark for this paper is 44.

QUESTION 2.1

A 4-month-old boy is admitted with diarrhoea since birth, tachypnoea and a seborrhoeic skin rash. There is no palpable lymphadenopathy. His family history is shown below.

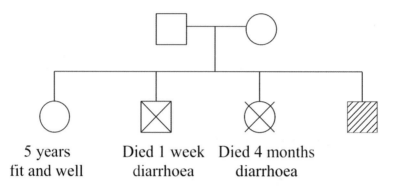

5 years   Died 1 week   Died 4 months
fit and well   diarrhoea   diarrhoea

Because of the tachypnoea and an oxygen saturation of 88%, he is given oxygen by mask; a chest X-ray and blood tests are taken. Despite iv amoxicillin and oral erythromycin the child fails to improve.

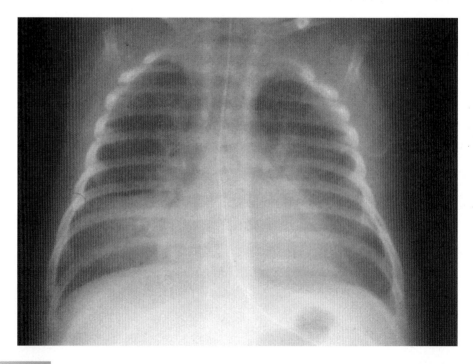

Investigations:

Hb: 11.0 g/dl
WBC: 5.1×10^9/litre (35% eosinophils)
Platelets: 255×10^9/litre
IgA absent
IgG low
IgM low

a) What is the underlying diagnosis? (1 mark)

Select ONE answer only

- [ ] A Isolated IgA deficiency
- [ ] B Bruton's hypogammaglobulinaemia
- [ ] C Human immunodeficiency virus
- [ ] D Severe combined immune deficiency
- [ ] E Wiscott–Aldrich syndrome

b) What is the most likely organism causing the pneumonia? (1 mark)

Select ONE answer only

- [ ] A *Streptococcus pneumoniae*
- [ ] B *Mycoplasma pneumoniae*
- [ ] C *Chlamydia psittaci*
- [ ] D *Pneumocystis jiroveci*
- [ ] E *Pseudomonas aeruginosa*

c) What is the treatment of choice for this child? (1 mark)

Select ONE answer only

- [ ] A Intravenous cephalosporin
- [ ] B Intravenous fluconazole
- [ ] C Intravenous macrolide
- [ ] D Oral co-trimoxazole
- [ ] E Intravenous co-trimoxazole

QUESTION 2.2

A 9-day-old baby is admitted with a 2-day history of diarrhoea and vomiting. He had an unremarkable perinatal history with birth weight 3.7 kg. Initially he had bottle fed well. Both parents recently had gastroenteritis. Whilst in hospital he is started on intravenous fluids as he continued to vomit.

Initial urine microscopy showed haematuria and he became oliguric during the course of the day. Ten hours after admission he has two short generalised convulsions. On examination he looks pale and clinically dehydrated. He dislikes abdominal examination, with screaming and drawing his legs up to his chest. A mass is palpable in the right hypochondrium. The rest of the examination is normal.

Investigations

Hb: 16 g/dl
WBC: 22.1 × 10⁹/litre (70% neutrophils)
Platelets: 35 × 10⁹/litre
Urea: 28 mmol/litre

a) What is the most likely diagnosis? (1 mark)

Select ONE answer only

- [ ] A Intussusception
- [ ] B Volvulus
- [ ] C Gastroenteritis and dehydration
- [ ] D Haemolytic uraemic syndrome
- [ ] E Necrotising enterocolitis
- [ ] F Renal vein thrombosis
- [ ] G Overwhelming urinary tract infection with septicaemia
- [ ] H GI malrotation

b) What is the most useful investigation to confirm diagnosis?
    (1 mark)

Select ONE answer only

- [ ] A Abdominal X-ray
- [ ] B GI contrast enema
- [ ] C Serum creatinine
- [ ] D Abdominal ultrasound scan
- [ ] E Blood culture

c) Give three possible causes for the convulsions in this case? (3 marks)

Select THREE answers only

- [ ] A Hypernatraemia
- [ ] B Hyponatraemia
- [ ] C Meningitis
- [ ] D Intracranial haemorrhage
- [ ] E Hypocalcaemia
- [ ] F Hypercalcaemia
- [ ] G Hypertension
- [ ] H Encephalitis
- [ ] I Hypoglycaemia

QUESTION 2.3

Consider the following X-ray.

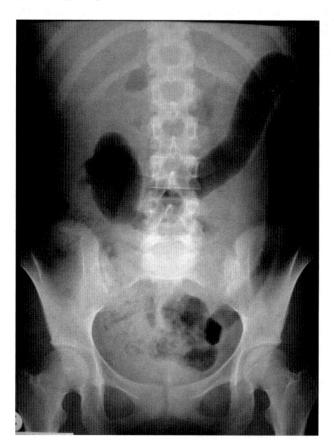

a) **What is the most likely diagnosis? (1 mark)**

Select ONE answer only

- [ ] A Crohn's disease
- [ ] B Hirschsprung's disease
- [ ] C Coeliac disease
- [ ] D Constipation
- [ ] E Ulcerative colitis

QUESTION 2.4

A 2-year-old boy presents with recurrent convulsions. He was born by forceps delivery at 2.4 kg. His development has been normal and his immunisations up to date. His parents are both 25 years old and well, although his father suffered from fits until the age of 3. The 4-year-old sister is well.

His first attack occurred 6 months ago following an upper respiratory tract infection associated with fever. Four more attacks have occurred, all in the early morning. The child is said to be irritable before breakfast and possibly a little unsteady on his feet. He is well in between attacks and takes phenobarbitone 30 mg bd. On examination he is alert and looks healthy. His height and weight are both below the 3rd centile. There is a 3 cm smooth hepatomegaly but otherwise examination is normal.

Investigations

Na:	138 mmol/litre
K:	4.5 mmol/litre
Urea:	4.0 mmol/litre
Ca:	2.25 mmol/litre
PO_4:	1.2 mmol/litre
Alkaline phosphatase:	800 IU
Fasting glucose:	1.6 mmol/litre
Fasting plasma:	ketones elevated
Post-prandial glucose:	4.8 mmol/litre
Hb:	11.9g/dl
WBC:	6.4×10^9/litre
Bone age:	18 months

a) What is the most likely diagnosis? (1 mark)

Select ONE answer only

- ☐ A Nesidioblastosis
- ☐ B Medium chain Acyl-Co-A dehydrogenase (MCAD) deficiency
- ☐ C Type I glycogen storage disease (glucose-6-phosphatase deficiency)
- ☐ D Glycogen synthetase deficiency
- ☐ E Ketotic hypoglycaemia

b) What investigation would you use to confirm the diagnosis?
(1 mark)

Select ONE answer only

- [ ] A Provocation fast
- [ ] B Urine reducing substance
- [ ] C Liver glycogen synthetase activity
- [ ] D Urinary organic acids
- [ ] E Electroencephalogram (EEG)

QUESTION 2.5

Consider the following criteria for withdrawal and withholding life-saving treatment.

A   The 'brain dead' child
B   The 'permanent vegetative' state
C   The 'no chance' situation
D   The 'no purpose' situation
E   The 'unbearable' situation

a)   Choose the most appropriate criteria from the list above for the following clinical situations. (1 mark each, total 5 marks). Each answer may be used once, more than once or not at all.

Select ONE answer only for each situation

- [ ] 1. A child with leukaemia, who has relapsed twice – doctors advise a further course of chemotherapy and total body irradiation followed by a second bone marrow transplant. The child does not want further treatment.
- [ ] 2. The degree of impairment or disability following recovery from meningitis would be so great that it is unreasonable to expect the child to bear it. The child is incapable of ever taking part in decisions regarding his or her care.
- [ ] 3. A child left in a state of unawareness of self and environment 12 months following a head injury.
- [ ] 4. A ventilated neonate with bilateral intraventricular haemorrhages with extensive haemorrhagic infarcts.
- [ ] 5. A 21-week gestation neonate born at 400 g whose parents want full intensive care.

QUESTION 2.6

A child is referred by his G.P. with the following features.

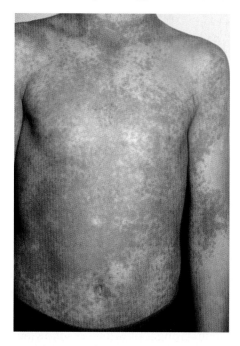

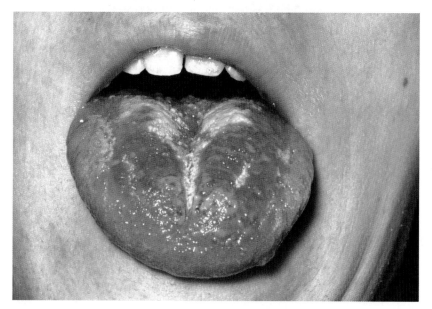

a) What is the most likely diagnosis? (1 mark)

Select ONE answer only

- ☐ A Kawasaki disease
- ☐ B Measles
- ☐ C Roseola
- ☐ D Rubella
- ☐ E Scarlet fever

QUESTION 2.7

A 6-year-old girl is being investigated for poor school performance. The school reports her to not be listening in class, and to have severe behavioural difficulties.

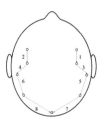
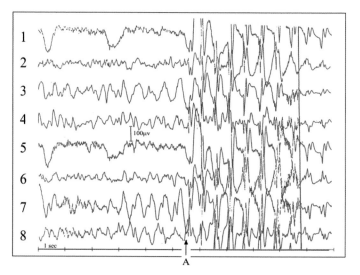

a) What is shown on the EEG? (1 mark)

Select ONE answer only

- ☐ A   Benign rolandic epilepsy
- ☐ B   Hypsarrhythmia
- ☐ C   Subacute sclerosing panencephalitis
- ☐ D   3-per-second spike and wave activity
- ☐ E   Encephalitis

b) What manoeuvre could have been performed at point A? (1 mark)

Select ONE answer only

- [ ] A Photostimulation
- [ ] B Lorazepam iv
- [ ] C Hyperventilation
- [ ] D Breath holding
- [ ] E Aciclovir iv

c) What further investigations would you perform before starting treatment? (1 mark)

Select ONE answer only

- [ ] A None
- [ ] B Sleep-deprived EEG
- [ ] C MRI scan
- [ ] D Amino acid screen
- [ ] E CT scan

QUESTION 2.8

A 10-month-old boy from Kenya is referred with failure to thrive. He weighs 4.1 kg and was apparently a normal baby. He is able to sit up if gently supported; he cannot yet crawl or pull himself to stand. He has a preference to reach with his left hand and demonstrates fine prehension. He babbles and coos but has no words.

a) Considering this child's development (3 marks)

Select THREE statements only

- ☐ A Normal gross motor development
- ☐ B Mildly delayed gross motor development
- ☐ C Severely delayed gross motor development
- ☐ D Normal fine motor development
- ☐ E Mildly delayed fine motor development
- ☐ F Severely delayed fine motor development
- ☐ G Normal speech and language development
- ☐ H Mildly delayed speech and language development
- ☐ I Severely delayed speech and language development

He has suffered recurrent otitis media despite antibiotic treatment.

Investigations

Hb:	8.9 g/dl
WBC:	16×10^9/litre
PMN:	50%
Lymphocytes:	40%
Monocytes:	6%
Eosinophils:	1%
ESR:	15 mm/hour
Sickle test:	negative
Albumin:	23 g/litre

Immunoglobulins:
   IgG: 410 IU/ml (35–115)
   IgM: 236 IU/ml (35–185)
   IgA: 96 IU/ml (10–65)

b) What is the probable diagnosis? (1 mark)

Select ONE answer only

- ☐ A Acquired immunodeficiency syndrome (AIDS)
- ☐ B Systemic onset juvenile idiopathic arthritis
- ☐ C Hyper IgM syndrome
- ☐ D Schwachmann–Diamond syndrome
- ☐ E Systemic lupus erythematosus

QUESTION 2.9

A teenage girl presents to casualty with the spreading rash shown.

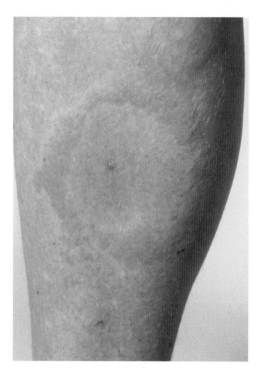

a) What is the rash? (1 mark)

Select ONE answer only

- [ ] A Erythema nodosum
- [ ] B Herald patch of pityriasis rosea
- [ ] C Erythema marginatum
- [ ] D Psoriasis
- [ ] E Erythema chronicum migrans

QUESTION 2.10

During the postnatal check a 1-day old baby is noted to be hypotonic with a poor Moro reflex. An ECG is taken.

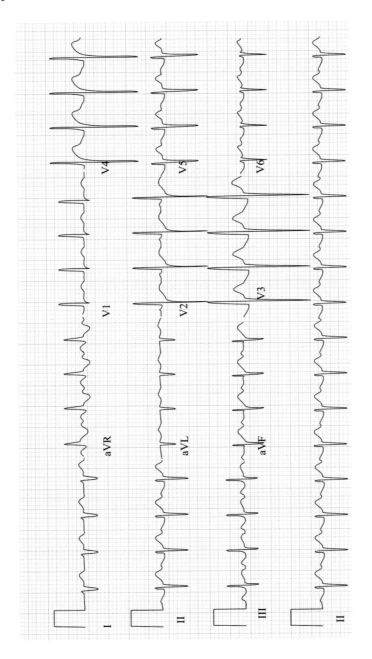

a)   What three findings are consistent with the ECG shown? (3 marks)

Select THREE answers only

- ☐ A   Neonatal RS progression
- ☐ B   P mitrale
- ☐ C   Prolonged PR interval
- ☐ D   Left bundle branch block
- ☐ E   Right bundle branch block
- ☐ F   Bifascicular block
- ☐ G   Left axis
- ☐ H   Superior axis
- ☐ I   Right axis

b)   What is the probable diagnosis? (1 mark)

Select ONE answer only

- ☐ A   Atrial septal defect
- ☐ B   Ebstein's anomaly
- ☐ C   Atrioventricular septal defect
- ☐ D   Tetralogy of Fallot
- ☐ E   Ventricular septal defect

QUESTION 2.11

A child with a 1-week history of febrile illness treated with ampicillin presents with mild neck stiffness and hemiplegia.

Cerebrospinal fluid
Protein: 0.8 g/litre
Glucose: 0.7 mmol/litre
WBC: 300 per mm³, 68% lymphocytes

Peripheral blood
Glucose: 5.5 mmol/litre
WBC: 15 × 10⁹/litre, 58% lymphocytes

a)   What is the diagnosis? (1 mark)

Select ONE answer only

☐ A Viral meningitis
☐ B Mumps encephalitis
☐ C Partially treated bacterial meningitis
☐ D Tuberculous meningitis
☐ E Herpes encephalitis

QUESTION 2.12

Consider the following photograph.

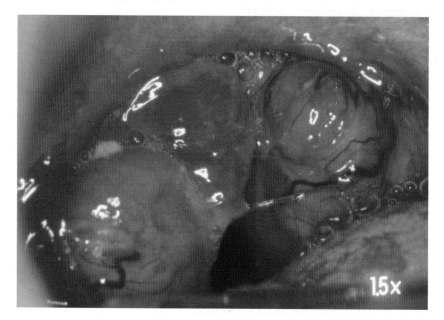

a) **What is the diagnosis? (1 mark)**

Select ONE answer only

- [ ] A   Quinsy
- [ ] B   Diphtheria
- [ ] C   Glandular fever
- [ ] D   Acute viral tonsillitis
- [ ] E   Acute bacterial tonsillitis

QUESTION 2.13

A 28-week preterm baby is being ventilated for respiratory distress syndrome. The baby is sedated, the ventilator is set at:

Rate 50 per minute
Pressure 20/3 cmH$_2$O
I:E ratio 1:1.5
FiO$_2$ 0.8

A set of arterial gases are taken:

pH:	7.15
PaO$_2$:	6.4 kPa
PaCO$_2$:	7.5 kPa
Base excess:	–7.1 mmol/litre

Consider the following ventilatory changes:

A Increase peak inspiratory pressure (PIP)
B Decrease peak inspiratory pressure (PIP)
C Increase positive end expiratory pressure (PEEP)
D Decrease positive end expiratory pressure (PEEP)
E Increase I:E ratio
F Decrease I:E ratio
G Increase rate

a) Choose the most appropriate method from the list above to achieve the following. (1 mark each, total 5 marks). Each answer may be used once, more than once or not at all.

Select ONE answer only for each situation

- [ ] 1. Increase oxygenation alone
- [ ] 2. Increase carbon dioxide elimination alone
- [ ] 3. Increase oxygenation and carbon dioxide elimination
- [ ] 4. Increase oxygenation, reduce carbon dioxide elimination
- [ ] 5. Reduce oxygenation, increase carbon dioxide elimination

QUESTION 2.14

The following MAG3 scan is taken from a child under investigation for hydronephrosis.

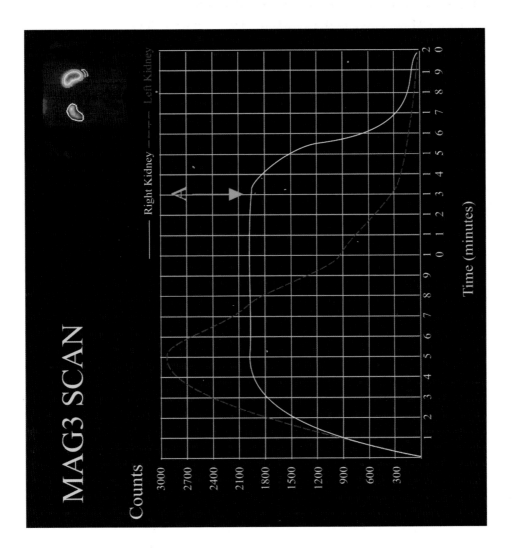

a) What features are seen on the MAG3? (2 marks)

Select TWO answers only

- [ ] A Left renal artery stenosis
- [ ] B Right renal artery stenosis
- [ ] C Left renal outflow obstruction
- [ ] D Right renal outflow obstruction
- [ ] E Left baggy collecting system
- [ ] F Right baggy collecting system
- [ ] G Reduced left differential function
- [ ] H Reduced right differential function
- [ ] I Right renal scarring
- [ ] J Right vesicoureteric reflux

b) What manoeuvre occurred at point 'A'? (1 mark)

Select ONE answer only

- [ ] A Bladder catheterisation
- [ ] B Bladder washout
- [ ] C Fluid bolus iv
- [ ] D Passing urine
- [ ] E Furosemide administration iv

QUESTION 2.15

Examine this blood film.

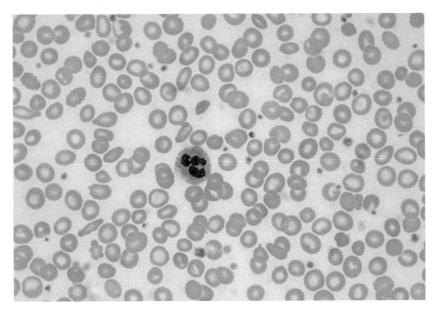

a)   What findings are present? (4 marks)

Select FOUR answers only

☐ A Microcytosis
☐ B Macrocytosis
☐ C Anisosytosis
☐ D Poikilocytosis
☐ E Hypersegmented neutrophils
☐ F Thrombocytopenia
☐ G Sickle cells
☐ H Leucopenia
☐ I   Nucleated red blood cells
☐ J Acanthocytes
☐ K Pencil cells
☐ L Schistocytes
☐ M Rouleaux formation

b) What is the most likely diagnosis? (1 mark)

Select ONE answer only

- ☐ A   Sideroblastic anaemia
- ☐ B   Acute lymphoblastic leukaemia
- ☐ C   Thalassaemia
- ☐ D   Iron deficiency anaemia
- ☐ E   Sickle cell anaemia

MRCPCH PART 2 EXAMINATION

Practice Exam 3

Answer all 15 questions in the allotted time (2½ hours). At the end of each question the value of that question is shown in brackets. The total mark for this paper is 44.

QUESTION 3.1

A 12-year-old schoolboy presents with lower back pain. It began 3 weeks ago during a school PE lesson. He initially stayed in bed but despite rest still complained of continual pain. He found walking painful and seemed unsteady on his feet. His throat has been sore for the past week and his appetite poor. Although he has no dysuria, he complains of frequency and occasional incontinence of urine.

On examination he looks unwell, and is pyrexial at 38°C. There are pale conjunctivae and there is a lesion on his left thigh as in the photograph.

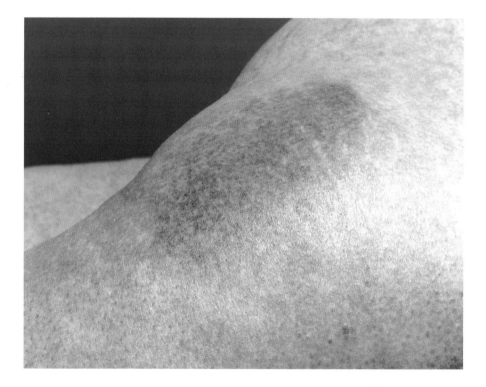

Examination of his throat reveals redness but no exudate. His back and neck are stiff with restricted movements. Neurological examination reveals increased tone in the legs and an absent right ankle jerk. Sensation over the dorsum of the right foot is reduced.

a) What is the underlying diagnosis? (1 mark)

Select ONE answer only

- ☐ A Guillain–Barré syndrome
- ☐ B Meningococcal meningitis
- ☐ C Acute lymphoblastic leukaemia
- ☐ D Infectious mononucleosis
- ☐ E Transverse myelitis

b) What investigations would be of most use to establish the diagnosis? (2 marks)

Select TWO answers only

- ☐ A Full blood count
- ☐ B MRI scan of the spine
- ☐ C Blood cultures
- ☐ D CT scan of the brain
- ☐ E Bone marrow aspirate
- ☐ F Monospot test
- ☐ G Throat swab

QUESTION 3.2

An 8-year-old boy with cystic fibrosis presents with gradual onset of generalised abdominal pain and bile-stained vomiting over the last 2 days.

On examination he is apyrexial but appears 5% dehydrated. His abdomen is moderately distended with generalised tenderness but no guarding. There is a firm mass palpable in the right iliac fossa.

a) What are the three most likely diagnoses? (3 marks)

Select THREE answers only

- [ ] A Distal intestinal obstruction syndrome
- [ ] B Pancreatitis
- [ ] C Gallstones
- [ ] D Ascending cholangitis
- [ ] E Appendix abscess
- [ ] F Intussusception
- [ ] G Constipation
- [ ] H Meconium ileus

b) What investigation would be most helpful? (1 mark)

Select ONE answer only

- [ ] A Abdominal ultrasound
- [ ] B Endoscopic retrograde cholecystopancreatogram (ERCP)
- [ ] C Contrast enema
- [ ] D Serum amylase
- [ ] E Abdominal X-ray

QUESTION 3.3

Consider the following X-ray.

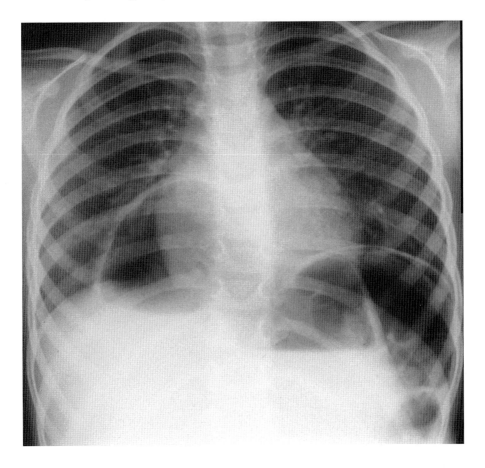

a. What is shown? (1 mark)

Select ONE answer only

- [ ] A Cystic adenomatoid malformation
- [ ] B Congenital emphysema
- [ ] C Pneumatocoele
- [ ] D Congenital diaphragmatic hernia
- [ ] E Pneumothorax

QUESTION 3.4

A 14-year-old girl presents with pain in the lower back and difficulty bending down for the last 3 days. She thinks her face is slightly swollen and feels weak in her arms and legs. Earlier in the day she had an episode of double vision lasting half an hour. At the age of 6 she suffered meningitis but made a complete recovery.

On examination she is not breathless or cyanosed. She has no neck stiffness and has an expressionless face. She is unable to close her eyes when asked. Neither can she lift her limbs off the couch. All limb reflexes are absent, the abdominal reflex is present and sensation to light touch is intact.

Investigations

Hb:	12.6 g/dl
WBC:	5.8 × 10⁹/litre
ESR:	7 mm/hour
Na:	134 mmol/litre
K:	5.2 mmol/litre
Urea:	5.5 mmol/litre
Creatine:	62 mmol/litre

a) What is the most likely diagnosis? (1 mark)

Select ONE answer only

- ☐ A Subacute sclerosing panencephalitis
- ☐ B Creutzfeld–Jakob disease
- ☐ C Guillain–Barré syndrome
- ☐ D Transverse myelitis
- ☐ E Viral encephalomyelitis

b) **What diagnostic investigations would you perform next? (1 mark)**

Select ONE answer only

- ☐ A Spirometry
- ☐ B MRI scan of the spine
- ☐ C Lumbar puncture
- ☐ D CT scan of the brain
- ☐ E Nerve conduction studies

c) **What should be used to monitor her progress? (1 mark)**

Select ONE answer only

- ☐ A Spirometry
- ☐ B MRI scan of the spine
- ☐ C Lumbar puncture
- ☐ D CT scan of the brain
- ☐ E Nerve conduction studies

QUESTION 3.5

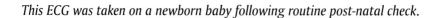

This ECG was taken on a newborn baby following routine post-natal check.

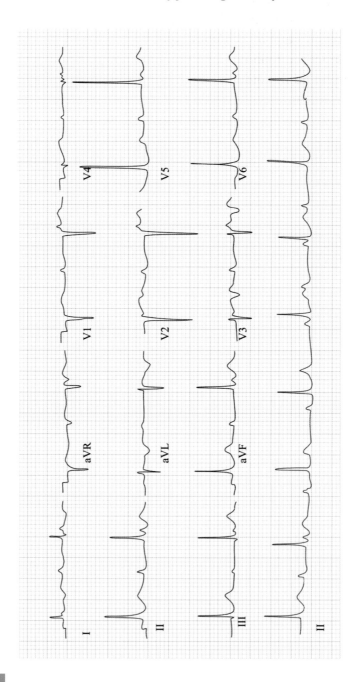

a) What diagnosis is consistent with the ECG shown? (1 mark)

Select ONE answer only

☐ A   1st degree heart block
☐ B   2nd degree heart block Mobitz type 1
☐ C   2nd degree heart block Mobitz type 2
☐ D   Bifasicular heart block
☐ E   Complete heart block

b) What is the most commonly associated maternal illness? (1 mark)

Select ONE answer only

☐ A   Rheumatoid arthritis
☐ B   Systemic lupus erythematosus
☐ C   Systemic sclerosis
☐ D   Dermatomyositis
☐ E   Polymyositis

QUESTION 3.6

The child shown in the photograph attends casualty complaining of the rash and severe abdominal pain.

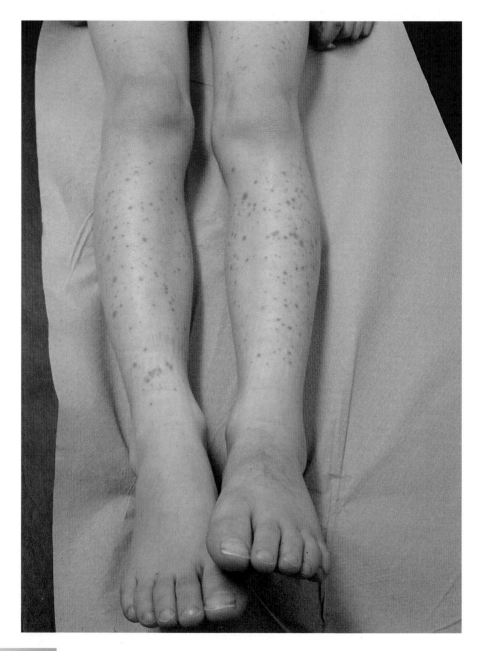

a) What would be the appropriate response? (1 mark)

Select ONE answer only

- ☐ A Reassure and discharge home
- ☐ B Prescribe laxatives
- ☐ C Discharge with regular analgesics
- ☐ D Prescribe a course of oral steroids
- ☐ E Arrange an abdominal ultrasound scan

QUESTION 3.7

Considering the following family tree of the boy affected with the condition shown.

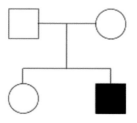

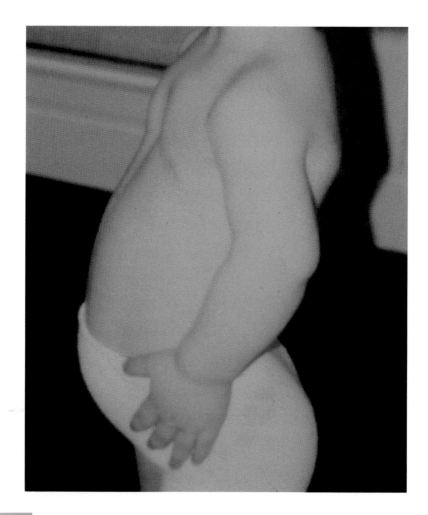

Consider the following list of probabilities.

A   Zero

B   < 1%

C   1%

D   5%

E   25%

F   50%

G   67%

H   100%

a)   Choose the most appropriate risk from the list above for the following situations (1 mark each, total 4 marks). Each answer may be used once, more than once or not at all.

Select ONE answer only for each situation

☐   1. What is the chance of a further child being affected?

☐   2. What is the risk of the sibling having an affected child?

☐   3. What is the chance that a male offspring of the boy will have the disease?

☐   4. What is the chance that a female offspring of the boy will have the disease?

QUESTION 3.8

A 13-year-old girl is brought for consultation by her mother who believes the girl is not growing. Assessment shows her weight to be increasing satisfactorily and her height to be below the third centile. Her height velocity is falling and she has not entered puberty. Her bone age is 8.28 years.

a) **What investigations would you consider next? (2 marks)**

Select TWO answers only

- A Full blood count
- B CT head
- C Thyroid function tests
- D Blood glucose
- E Chromosomes
- F Renal function tests
- G Isotope thyroid scan

Combined pituitary function tests are shown below:

Time (mins)	0	20	30	60	90	120
Glucose mmol/litre	4.1	0.9	2.1	6.5	8.1	8.7
Cortisol nmol/litre	337	797	868	710	640	
GH mU/litre	0.9	1.4	11.6	4.5	1.0	
TSH mU/litre	>60	59	>60			

b) **What is the diagnosis? (1 mark)**

Select ONE answer only

- A Growth hormone deficiency
- B Primary hypothyroidism
- C Constitutional delay in growth and puberty
- D Turner's syndrome
- E Secondary hypothyroidism

QUESTION 3.9

Consider the following photograph.

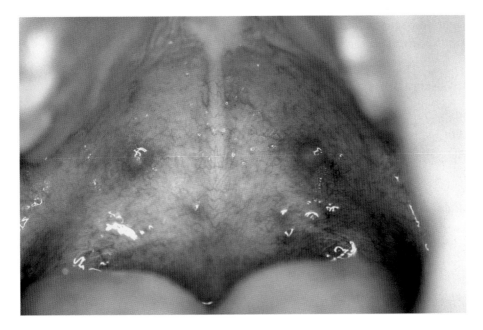

a) **What is the cause of the lesions shown? (1 mark)**

Select ONE answer only

- [ ] A Varicella zoster
- [ ] B Coxsackie virus
- [ ] C Herpes simplex
- [ ] D Adenovirus
- [ ] E *Staphylococcus aureus*

QUESTION 3.10

A 5-month-old infant presents with a vague history of malaise, lethargy and fever for 2 weeks. On examination he has a macular rash over his body, his hands are slightly oedematous and peeling. His tonsils are enlarged and he has some large lymph nodes in his neck.

Investigations

Hb:	11.1 g/dl
WBC:	24.0 × 10⁹/litre
Platelets:	680 × 10⁹/litre
Na:	133 mmol/litre
K:	4.5 mmol/litre
HCO₃:	18 mmol/litre
Urea:	3.5 mmol/litre

a) What is the most important differential diagnosis? (1 mark)

Select ONE answer only

☐ A Measles
☐ B Scarlet fever
☐ C Staphylococcal scalded skin syndrome
☐ D Toxic epidermolysis necrolysis
☐ E Kawasaki's disease

b) What investigations would be of most use to establish the diagnosis? (3 marks)

Select THREE answers only

☐ A Serial full blood counts
☐ B Serological testing
☐ C Blood cultures
☐ D Throat swab
☐ E ASO titre
☐ F Monospot test
☐ G Differential white blood count

c) What immediate management should be commenced? (1 mark)

Select ONE answer only

☐ A Immunoglobulin iv
☐ B Flucloxacillin iv
☐ C Hydrocortisone iv
☐ D Aciclovir iv
☐ E Penicillin iv

QUESTION 3.11

Consider the following EEG.

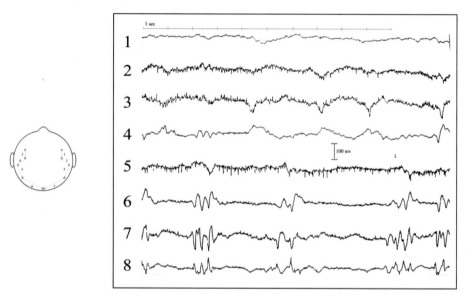

a) What diagnosis would be compatible? (1 mark)

Select ONE answer only

☐ A Subacute sclerosing panencephalitis
☐ B Encephalitis
☐ C Infantile spasms
☐ D Benign rolandic epilepsy
☐ E Simple absence seizures

b) Name one cause (1 mark)

Select ONE answer only

☐ A Measles
☐ B Tuberous sclerosis
☐ C Von Hippel–Lindau syndrome
☐ D Congenital rubella
☐ E Herpes simplex virus

QUESTION 3.12

Consider the following photo.

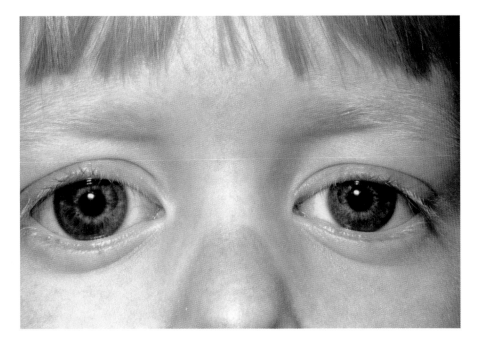

a) What is the cause of the appearance shown? (1 mark)

Select ONE answer only

- [ ] A Congenital glaucoma
- [ ] B Wilson's disease
- [ ] C CHARGE association
- [ ] D Familial dyslipidaemia
- [ ] E Horner's syndrome

QUESTION 3.13

A well 8-week-old baby is referred because of pallor noticed in a routine 6-week development clinic. This is the mother's second child and the neonatal period was uneventful.

Investigations

Mothers blood group: A NEG
Cord blood:

    Hb: 16.2 g/dl
    WBC: 10.1 × 10⁹/litre
    Platelets: 261 × 10⁹/litre
    Group   O POS
    DAT: NEG

At 8 weeks

    Hb: 5.1 g/dl
    WBC: 12.4 × 10⁹/litre
    Platelets: 321 × 10⁹/litre

a) What investigations would be of most use? (3 marks)

Select THREE answers only

- [ ] A   Blood film
- [ ] B   Father's blood group
- [ ] C   Bone marrow aspiration
- [ ] D   Repeat DAT
- [ ] E   Indirect antiglobulin test
- [ ] F   Red cell enzyme levels
- [ ] G   Reticulocyte count
- [ ] H   Atypical antibody panel
- [ ] I   Haptoglobin levels
- [ ] J   Haemoglobin electrophoresis
- [ ] K   Monospot test

b) What is the most likely diagnosis? (1 mark)

Select ONE answer only

- ☐ A Rhesus haemolytic disease of the newborn
- ☐ B Thalassaemia
- ☐ C Fanconi's anaemia
- ☐ D Pyruvate kinase deficiency
- ☐ E Diamond–Blackfan syndrome

QUESTION 3.14

Consider the following list of developmental milestones.

A   Cuts a strip off the edge of a square of paper
B   Rides a tricycle
C   Uses a knife and fork at the table
D   Builds a tower of 8 bricks
E   Runs and kicks a ball
F   Able to undress
G   Stands on one foot for 6 seconds
H   Draws a recognisable man
I   Knows first name

a) Choose the appropriate assessment for the following milestones. (1 mark each, total 9 marks). Each answer may be used once, more than once or not at all.

Select ONE answer only for each situation

☐ 1. Personal and social skill age 3
☐ 2. Eye hand coordination age 3
☐ 3. Locomotor milestone age 3
☐ 4. Personal and social skill age 4
☐ 5. Eye hand coordination age 4
☐ 6. Locomotor milestone age 4
☐ 7. Personal and social skill age 5
☐ 8. Eye hand coordination age 5
☐ 9. Locomotor milestone age 5

QUESTION 3.15

The following was seen on examination of the ear of a pyrexial child.

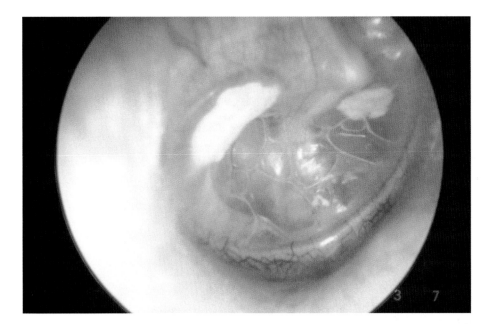

a) What would be the most appropriate action? (1 mark)

Select ONE answer only

- ☐ A   Prescribe a 5-day course of antibiotics
- ☐ B   Refer to an ENT surgeon
- ☐ C   Reassure parents, and discharge with antipyretics
- ☐ D   Prescribe a 7-day course of antibiotics
- ☐ E   Obtain a CT scan

MRCPCH PART 2 EXAMINATION

Practice Exam 4

Answer all 15 questions in the allotted time (2½ hours). At the end of each question the value of that question is shown in brackets. The total mark for this paper is 34.

QUESTION 4.1

A 10-week-old girl presents to A&E with abdominal distension. She was born in India at 38 weeks (birth weight 2.3 kg) and came to England at 3 weeks of age. Her parents feel that she has been constipated.

On examination she appears pale and unwell with a rash on her trunk as shown. Her weight is 3.23 kg, temperature 36.4°C, pulse 110 and respiratory rate 32 breaths per minute. She is floppy with no head control; her parents have never seen her smile. Her abdomen is generally distended and her liver is palpable 1 cm below the costal margin. An abdominal X-ray is obtained.

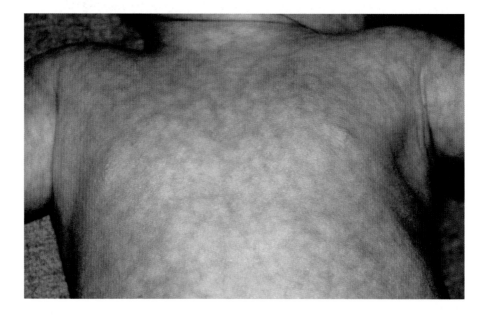

Other investigations are performed:

Hb: 10.2 g/dl
WBC: 8.3 × 10⁹/litre
Platelets: 450 × 10⁹/litre
Chest X-ray: normal
Urinalysis: normal

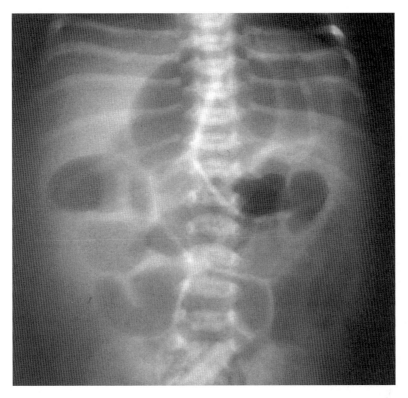

a) **What is the most likely cause of the abdominal distension: (1 mark)**

Select ONE answer only

☐ A Constipation
☐ B Sepsis and paralytic ileus
☐ C Organomegaly
☐ D Hirschsprung's disease
☐ E Distal intestinal obstruction syndrome (meconium ileus equivalent)

b) **What is the most likely underlying disorder: (1 mark)**

Select ONE answer only

☐ A Congenital hypothyroidism
☐ B Group B streptococcus
☐ C Phenylketonuria
☐ D McCune–Albright syndrome
☐ E Cystic fibrosis

QUESTION 4.2

A 15-year-old girl with known complex congenital heart disease is referred to the paediatrician by her general practitioner. Two weeks previously she had complained of increasing shortness of breath and was noticed to have an irregular pulse. She is now experiencing chest pain and has coughed up blood-stained sputum. She had a repair of her heart defect at the age of 18 months and has had regular follow-up since.

On examination she is cyanosed, has a loud second heart sound and both systolic and diastolic murmurs. Her blood pressure and the rest of her physical examination are normal.

Consider the following diagnoses:

A   Pulmonary hypertension
B   Bacterial endocarditis
C   Atrial fibrillation
D   Mitral valve rupture
E   Pulmonary embolism
F   Myocardial infarction
G   Aortic dissection
H   Patch detachment
I   Eisenmenger's syndrome

a) Choose the most likely diagnosis for the following: (1 mark each, total 3 marks). Each answer may be used once, more than once or not at all.

Select ONE answer only for each situation

☐ 1. What complication of the original lesion has occurred?
☐ 2. What has precipitated the recent deterioration?
☐ 3. What is the most likely cause of the chest pain?

QUESTION 4.3

This child is referred to A&E:

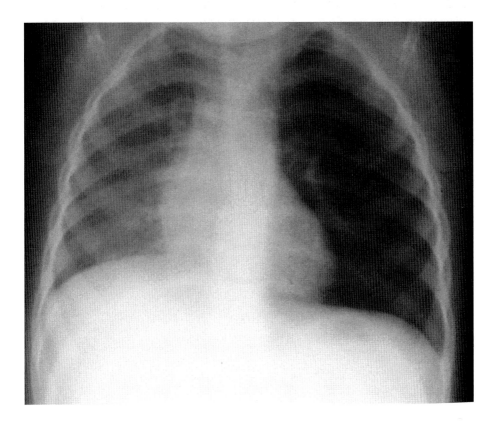

a) What is the diagnosis? (1 mark)

Select ONE answer only

☐ A Right sided pneumonia
☐ B Left pneumothorax
☐ C Left tension pneumothorax
☐ D Foreign body right main bronchus
☐ E Foreign body left main bronchus

QUESTION 4.4

Considering the following family tree.

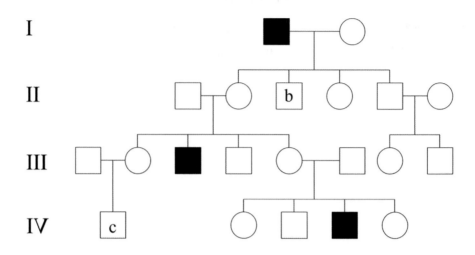

I

II

III

IV

a)   **What best describes the pattern of inheritance shown? (1 mark)**

Select ONE answer only

☐ A Autosomal dominant
☐ B Autosomal recessive
☐ C X-linked dominant
☐ D X-linked recessive
☐ E Mitochondrial

Consider the following list of probabilities.

☐ A Zero
☐ B < 1%
☐ C 1%
☐ D 5%
☐ E 25%
☐ F 50%
☐ G 67%
☐ H 100%

b) Choose the most appropriate risk from the list above for the following situations. (1 mark each, total 2 marks). Each answer may be used once, more than once or not at all.

Select ONE answer only for each situation

☐ 1. What is the chance of II_3 (b) being a carrier?
☐ 2. What is the chance of IV_1 (c) having the disease?

QUESTION 4.5

A previously bright 9-year-old girl, recently arrived in the UK from Boston, USA, is noted by her teachers to be falling behind academically. Her mother reports that she frequently drops her knife and fork and has recently noticed intermittent jerking of her arms and legs. An EEG/EMG is obtained.

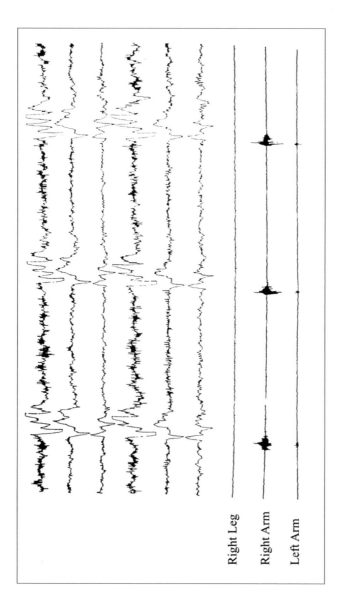

a) What is the diagnosis? (1 mark)

Select ONE answer only

- ☐ A Friedreich's ataxia
- ☐ B Subacute sclerosing panencephalitis
- ☐ C Hereditary sensory and motor neuropathy
- ☐ D Spinal muscular atrophy
- ☐ E Creutzfeld–Jakob disease

b) How can this be confirmed? (1 mark)

Select ONE answer only

- ☐ A Brain biopsy
- ☐ B CSF serology
- ☐ C FISH studies
- ☐ D Chromosome analysis
- ☐ E Muscle biopsy

QUESTION 4.6

This child is referred to A&E:

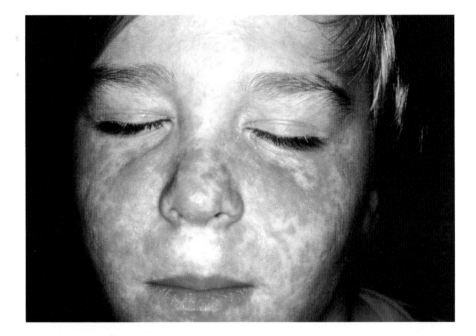

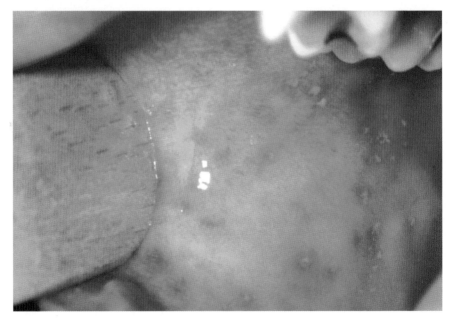

a) What is the diagnosis? (1 mark)

Select ONE answer only

- ☐ A Kawasaki's disease
- ☐ B Measles
- ☐ C Scarlet fever
- ☐ D Rubella
- ☐ E Parvovirus B19 infection

QUESTION 4.7

Examine this audiogram of a 10-year-old who had meningitis aged 3 years.

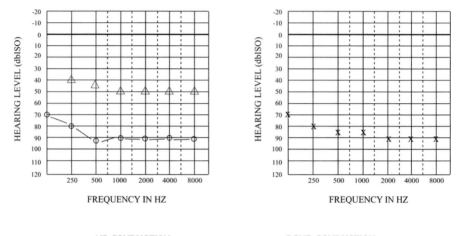

AIR CONDUCTION

o RIGHT   x LEFT

BONE CONDUCTION

△ UNMASKED (RIGHT OR LEFT)

a)   What abnormality is revealed? (1 mark)

Select ONE answer only

☐ A   Left moderate conductive hearing loss
☐ B   Left severe conductive hearing loss
☐ C   Left severe sensorineural hearing loss
☐ D   Right moderate conductive hearing loss
☐ E   Right severe conductive hearing loss
☐ F   Right severe sensorineural hearing loss
☐ G   Bilateral moderate conductive hearing loss
☐ H   Bilateral moderate sensorineural hearing loss
☐ I   Bilateral severe conductive hearing loss
☐ J   Bilateral severe sensorineural hearing loss

b) Suggest the most likely organism. (1 mark)

Select ONE answer only

- ☐ A *Meningococcus*
- ☐ B *Haemophilus influenza* B
- ☐ C *Streptococcus pneumoniae*
- ☐ D *Staphylococcus aureus*
- ☐ E *Klebsiella*

QUESTION 4.8

Following a normal postnatal check a baby girl becomes unwell on the postnatal ward day 3. The following cardiac catheter data is obtained.

Site	O$_2$ Saturation (%)	Pressure (mmHg)
SVC	55	8
RA	55	8
RV	75	80/8
PA	75	80/50
LA	91	12
LV	91	80/20
Abdominal aorta	85	55/45

a) **What three abnormalities are present? (3 marks)**

Select THREE answers only

☐ A Atrial septal defect
☐ B Ventricular septal defect with left-to-right shunting
☐ C Ventricular septal defect with right-to-left shunting
☐ D Right ventricular outflow obstruction
☐ E Patent ductus arteriosus with right-to-left shunting
☐ F Patent ductus arteriosus with left-to-right shunting
☐ G Coarctation of the aorta
☐ H Transposition of the great arteries

b) **What emergency treatment might this infant require? (1 mark)**

Select ONE answer only

☐ A Balloon atrial septostomy
☐ B Blalock–Taussig shunt
☐ C Intravenous prostacyclin
☐ D Intravenous prostaglandin
☐ E Ligation of ductus arteriosus

QUESTION 4.9

Consider the following appearance.

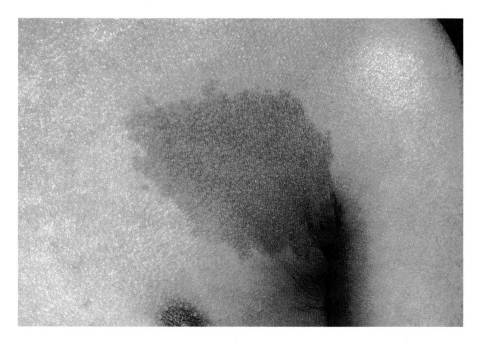

a) **What conditions are associated with this finding? (4 marks)**

Select FOUR answers only

- [ ] A Neurofibromatosis type I
- [ ] B Sturge–Weber syndrome
- [ ] C Phaeochromocytoma
- [ ] D Von Hippel–Lindau disease
- [ ] E McCune–Albright syndrome
- [ ] F Histiocytosis X
- [ ] G Sarcoidosis
- [ ] H Tuberous sclerosis
- [ ] I Nesidioblastosis
- [ ] J Systemic lupus erythematosus
- [ ] K Horner's syndrome
- [ ] L Fanconi anaemia

QUESTION 4.10

A 14-year-old boy with recent onset of bilateral facial palsy following a febrile illness has the following blood count.

Hb:	11.2 g/dl
MCV:	92 fl
MCH:	32 pg
MCHC:	34 g/dl
Reticulocytes:	5.7%
WBC:	16.2×10^9/litre
PMN:	49%
Lymphocytes:	51%
Platelets:	68×10^9/litre
ESR:	27 mm/hour

Blood film: atypical cells, spherocytes, and agglutination

a) What is the underlying diagnosis? (1 mark)

Select ONE answer only

- [ ] A Epstein–Barr virus
- [ ] B Mycoplasma
- [ ] C Brucellosis
- [ ] D Lyme disease
- [ ] E Malaria

b) What diagnostic test should be performed? (1 mark)

Select ONE answer only

- [ ] A Blood cultures
- [ ] B *Mycoplasma* serology
- [ ] C Monospot test
- [ ] D Thick and thin blood films
- [ ] E Osmotic fragility test

QUESTION 4.11

A 5-year-old girl presents to the outpatients department with a 6-month history of irritability, lethargy and low grade fevers. Her gait became waddling and her mother noticed she had difficulty climbing stairs. She developed a pink-purple rash over her face, eyelids and limbs.

Investigations

Hb:	10.3 g/dl
ESR:	22 mm/hour
CRP:	< 5 mg/litre
CK:	380 iu/litre
ANA:	positive
Rheumatoid factor:	negative

a) **What is the underlying diagnosis? (1 mark)**

Select ONE answer only

- [ ] A Polymyositis
- [ ] B Systemic lupus erythematosus
- [ ] C Dermatomyositis
- [ ] D Systemic onset juvenile idiopathic arthritis
- [ ] E Juvenile onset rheumatoid arthritis

b) **Suggest two confirmatory diagnostic tests. (2 marks)**

Select TWO answers only

- [ ] A Anti-double stranded DNA antibodies
- [ ] B Anti-Ro/La antibodies
- [ ] C Anti-smooth muscle antibodies
- [ ] D Renal biopsy
- [ ] E Skin biopsy
- [ ] F Muscle biopsy
- [ ] G EEG
- [ ] H EMG
- [ ] I ECG

c) What is the initial treatment? (1 mark)

Select ONE answer only

☐ A Methotrexate
☐ B Prednisolone
☐ C Ciclosporin
☐ D Azathioprine
☐ E Intravenous immunoglobulin

QUESTION 4.12

Consider the following appearance.

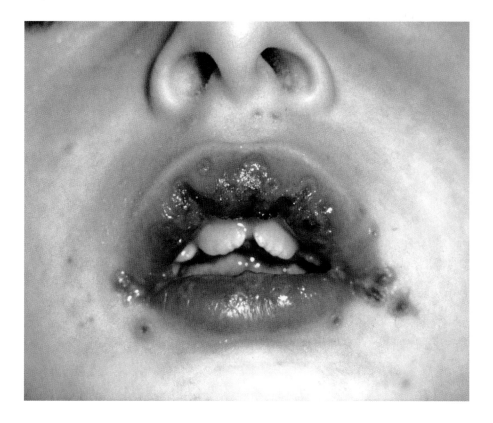

a) What is the diagnosis? (1 mark)

Select ONE answer only

- ☐ A Coxsackie virus (hand, foot and mouth disease)
- ☐ B Primary herpes gingivostomatitis
- ☐ C Stevens–Johnson syndrome
- ☐ D Varicella zoster
- ☐ E Toxic epidermolysis necrolysis

QUESTION 4.13

A baby boy aged 6 months is readmitted into hospital. He had spent the first 6 weeks in hospital because of a ventricular septal defect with associated heart failure. He was treated with furosemide and spironolactone and his condition improved before discharge.

At home feeding was always difficult until he started solid food at which time he stopped being breathless with feeds. At 3 months of age he developed diarrhoea, described as loose and foul smelling, up to 5 times a day.

On admission the baby looks tired, miserable and irritable. He is on furosemide 2mg bd and spironolactone 2.5mg bd. His weight is charted below.

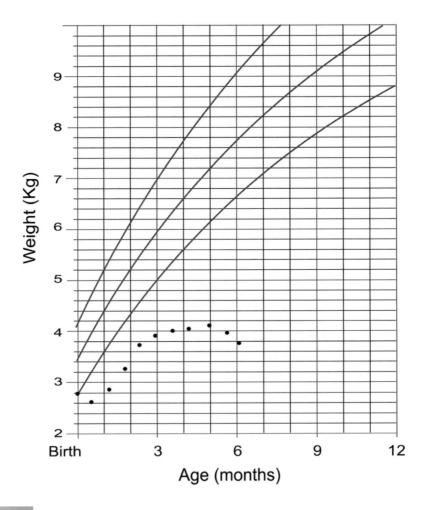

On examination his abdomen is slightly distended with a liver palpable 1cm below the costal margin. Examination of other systems is normal. Whilst in hospital he continues to have foul smelling, loose stools. Stool culture sent previously by the GP is negative.

Investigations

Hb:	10.3 g/dl
ESR:	9 mm/hour
CRP:	< 5 mg/litre
Urea:	6.3
Na:	147 mmol/litre
K:	3.1 mmol/litre
Creatinine:	37 μmol/litre

a) What is the cause of the failure to thrive? (1 mark)

Select ONE answer only

☐ A   Coeliac disease
☐ B   Congenital heart disease
☐ C   Crohn's disease
☐ D   Cow's milk protein intolerance
☐ E   Primary lactose intolerance

b) What is the best confirmatory diagnostic test (1 mark)

Select ONE answer only

☐ A   Echocardiogram
☐ B   Upper GI contrast study
☐ C   Upper GI endoscopy and biopsy
☐ D   Lower GI contrast study
☐ E   Stool reducing substance

QUESTION 4.14

An 11-year-old boy with cystic fibrosis complains of wheeze on exertion. Lung function tests are performed before and 20 minutes after nebulised salbutamol 5 mg.

	Pre	Post	Expected
Forced vital capacity (l)	1.7	1.8	2.1
FEV$_1$ (l)	1.0	1.5	1.81
Residual volume (l)	1.1	0.9	0.75
Total lung capacity (l)	3.3	3.1	3.0

a) What two abnormalities do these results show? (2 marks)

Select TWO answers only

- [ ] A Reversible obstructive airways disease
- [ ] B Non-reversible restrictive airways disease
- [ ] C Asthma
- [ ] D Reduced FEV$_1$/FVC after bronchodilation
- [ ] E Non-reversible obstructive airways disease
- [ ] F Reversible restrictive airways disease
- [ ] G Increased residual volume

QUESTION 4.15

Consider the following appearance.

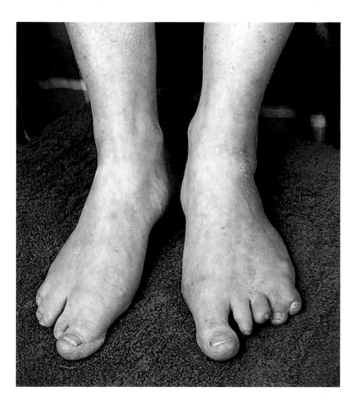

a) What is the diagnosis? (1 mark)

Select ONE answer only

- [ ] A Toxic epidermolysis necrolysis
- [ ] B TAR syndrome
- [ ] C Focal dermal hypoplasia syndrome
- [ ] D EEC syndrome
- [ ] E Naegeli–Franceschetti–Jadassohn syndrome.

MRCPCH PART 2 EXAMINATION

Practice Exam 5

Answer all 15 questions in the allotted time (2½ hours). At the end of each question the value of that question is shown in brackets. The total mark for this paper is 47.

QUESTION 5.1

A 6-year-old girl presents with cough, fever and mild respiratory distress. A chest X-ray is taken.

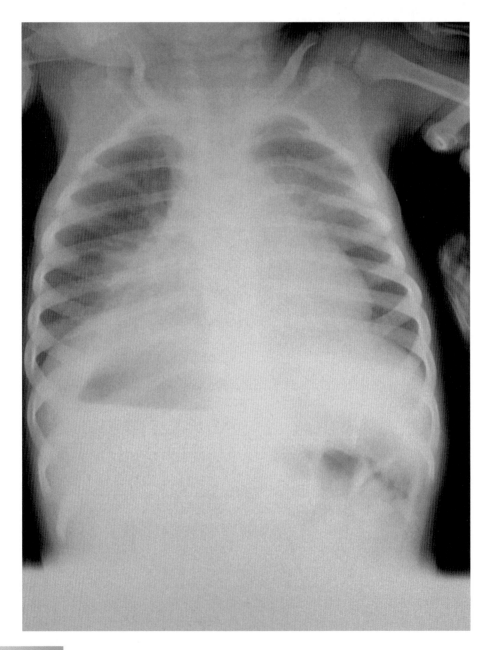

a) What best describes the X-ray appearance? (1 mark)

Select ONE answer only

- ☐ A Right lower lobe consolidation
- ☐ B Right lower lobe consolidation with collapse
- ☐ C Right middle lobe consolidation
- ☐ D Right middle lobe consolidation with collapse
- ☐ E Right pleural effusion
- ☐ F Right pleural effusion with middle lobe consolidation
- ☐ G Right pleural effusion with lower lobe consolidation

She is admitted to hospital and treated with intravenous antibiotics. Her condition responds well and she is discharged after 6 days. In her first 6 years of life she has had four episodes of pneumonia, one also on the right and others in different sites. Her first episode was at 18 months. Between episodes she is active and thriving.

She was born at 39 weeks and spent 12 hours on SCBU with unexplained tachypnoea. This settled, a septic screen was negative and she was returned to her mother.

When she was 3 years of age, community screening revealed a hearing loss, which was due to bilateral serous otitis media requiring grommets.

b) What three diagnostic investigations would you perform next? (3 marks)

Select THREE answers only

- ☐ A Immunoglobulins
- ☐ B Bronchoscopy and bronchoalveolar lavage
- ☐ C Ultrasound of the chest
- ☐ D CT scan of the chest
- ☐ E Blood culture
- ☐ F Sweat test
- ☐ G Mantoux test
- ☐ H Nasal brushings

c) What is the most likely diagnosis? (1 mark)

Select ONE answer only

- ☐ A Cystic fibrosis
- ☐ B Primary ciliary dyskinesia
- ☐ C Hyper-IgM syndrome
- ☐ D Cystic adenomatoid malformation
- ☐ E Common variable immunodeficiency

QUESTION 5.2

Consider the following family tree of two families with sensorineural deafness.

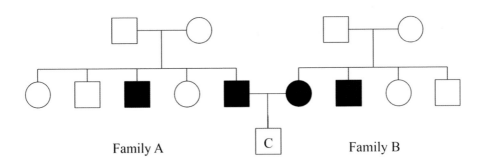

Family A   C   Family B

Now consider the following list of methods of inheritance.

A   Autosomal dominant

B   Autosomal recessive

C   X-linked dominant

D   X-linked recessive

E   Mitochondrial

a)   From the list above, what best describes the pattern of inheritance in family A? (1 mark)

Select ONE answer only

☐

b)   From the list above, what best describes the pattern of inheritance in family B? (1 mark)

Select ONE answer only

☐

c) What is the probability of the offspring 'c' having normal hearing? (1 mark)

Select ONE answer only

☐ A < 5%

☐ B 5%

☐ C 50%

☐ D 75%

☐ E > 95 %

QUESTION 5.3

Consider the following X-ray.

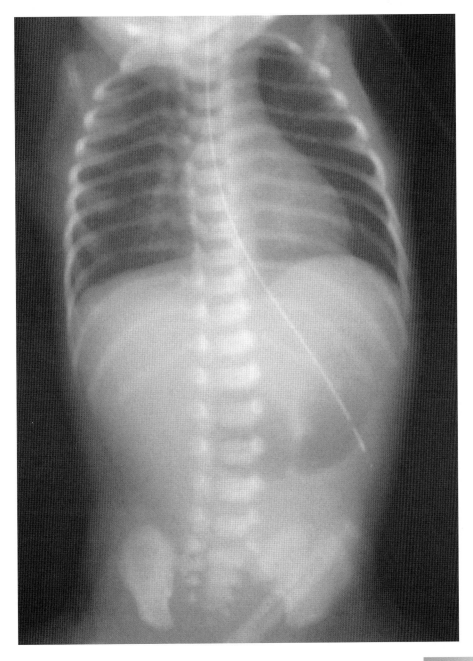

a) What is the diagnosis? (1 mark)

Select ONE answer only

☐ A   Duodenal atresia
☐ B   Hirschsprung's disease
☐ C   Jejunal atresia
☐ D   Intussusception
☐ E   Duodenal stenosis

QUESTION 5.4

A 13-year-old African boy known to have sickle cell disease presents with a 2-day history of intermittent abdominal pain. He has been admitted on many occasions with painful crises and in the last 2 years has required two exchange transfusions for severe sickle chest syndrome. When last seen in clinic he was well; his Hb was 8.1 g/dl and he was taking regular folic acid and penicillin.

Two days previously, after breakfast he suddenly felt a sharp abdominal pain, which made him bend double and later, feel nauseated. The pain settled for the rest of the day and he slept well. He was well the following day at school until the afternoon when the pain began again. It was present on admission to hospital but subsequently settled.

On examination he is quite a thin boy, and is apyrexial. Sclerae are mildly jaundiced, abdomen soft and the liver palpable 1 cm below the costal margin. He is tender in the epigastric region and right hypochondrium. The bowel sounds are normal.

Investigations

Hb:	8.0 g/dl
WBC:	11.4×10^9/litre
Platelets:	420×10^9/litre
Na:	131 mmol/litre
K:	4.0 mmol/litre

a) Give the most likely explanation for his symptoms. (1 mark)

Select ONE answer only

- [ ] A Girdle syndrome
- [ ] B Acute pancreatitis
- [ ] C Acute cholecystitis
- [ ] D Hepatic sequestration
- [ ] E Biliary colic

b) What one diagnostic investigation would you perform next?
     (1 mark)

Select ONE answer only

☐ A Abdominal ultrasound
☐ B Abdominal CT scan
☐ C Contrast enema
☐ D Abdominal X-ray
☐ E Serum amylase

QUESTION 5.5

Consider this age list with regard to developmental milestones.

A   1 year
B   2 years
C   3 years
D   4 years
E   5 years
F   6 years
G   7 years
H   8 years

a)   Choose the appropriate age for the following (1 mark each, total 9 marks). Each answer may be used once, more than once or not at all.

Select ONE answer only for each situation

☐   1. Copies a circle
☐   2. Able to put on own shoes and socks
☐   3. Knows first name

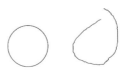

☐   4. Draws a triangle
☐   5. Builds a tower of 6 bricks

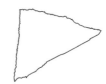

☐   6. Draws a house
☐   7. Runs downstairs
☐   8. Stands alone
☐   9. Bounces and catches a ball

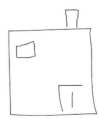

QUESTION 5.6

A 5-year-old child under investigation for recent onset failure to thrive develops the following painful lesions.

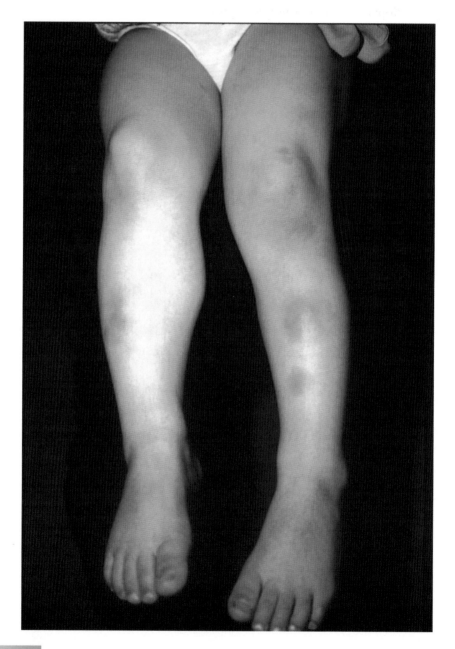

a) What is most likely diagnosis? (1 mark)

Select ONE answer only

- ☐ A Non-accidental injury
- ☐ B Erythema nodosum
- ☐ C Idiopathic thrombocytopenia purpura
- ☐ D Acute lymphoblastic leukaemia
- ☐ E Henoch-Schönlein purpura

QUESTION 5.7

The following cardiac catheter data are obtained from a 2-day-old infant.

Site	O_2 saturation (%)	Pressure (mmHg)
SVC	63	8
IVC	62	
RA	62	mean 4
RV	62	96/5
PA	61	24/5
PV	95	mean 4
LA	80	mean 4
LV	83	90/4
Femoral artery	83	90/55

a) **What three abnormalities are present? (3 marks)**

Select THREE answers only

☐ A Right-to-left shunting at the atrial level
☐ B Left-to-right shunting at the ventricular level
☐ C Critical aortic stenosis
☐ D Critical pulmonary stenosis
☐ E Patent ductus arteriosus with right-to-left shunting
☐ F Patent ductus arteriosus with left-to-right shunting
☐ G Coarctation of the aorta
☐ H Transposition of the great arteries

b) **What emergency treatment does this infant require? (1 mark)**

Select ONE answer only

☐ A Balloon atrial septostomy
☐ B Blalock–Taussig shunt
☐ C Intravenous prostacyclin
☐ D Intravenous prostaglandin
☐ E Ligation of ductus arteriosus

c) What definitive treatment will be required? (1 mark)

Select ONE answer only

- ☐ A Closure of an atrial septal defect
- ☐ B Closure of a ventricular septal defect
- ☐ C Arterial switch procedure
- ☐ D Balloon valvular dilatation
- ☐ E Pulmonary artery banding

QUESTION 5.8

Consider the following ECG.

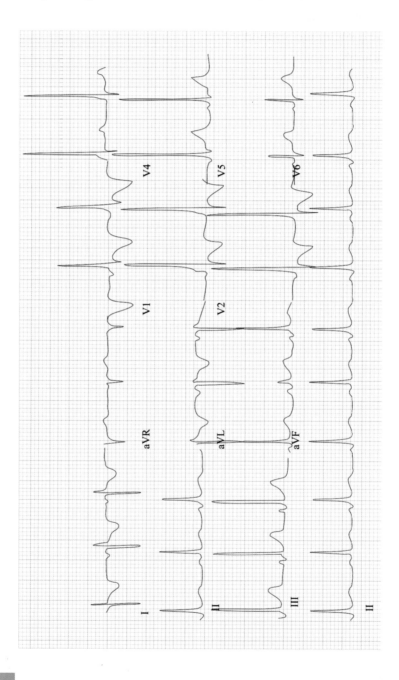

a) What two abnormalities are shown? (2 marks)

Select TWO answers only

☐ A   1st degree heart block
☐ B   Short PR interval
☐ C   Left ventricular hypertrophy
☐ D   δ wave
☐ E   Prolonged QT interval
☐ F   Right ventricular hypertrophy
☐ G   λ wave
☐ H   Q on T syndrome

b) What is the associated arrhythmia? (1 mark)

Select ONE answer only

☐ A   Ventricular tachycardia
☐ B   Junctional tachycardia
☐ C   Re-entry tachycardia
☐ D   Torsades de pointes
☐ E   Atrial fibrillation

QUESTION 5.9

Following a holiday in the Far East, a 14-year-old girl presents with the following skin lesions.

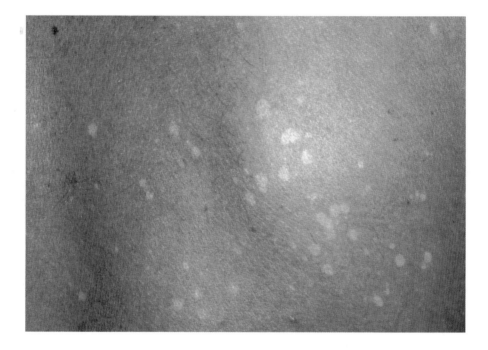

a) **What is most likely diagnosis? (1 mark)**

Select ONE answer only

- ☐ A Candida infection
- ☐ B Eczema
- ☐ C Staphylococcal infection
- ☐ D Pityriasis versicolor
- ☐ E Vitiligo

QUESTION 5.10

A 10-year-old girl presented with an intracranial tumour at the age of 9. She was treated with cranial radiotherapy. Subsequently she failed to grow.

Investigations

Thyroxine   58 nmol/litre

Insulin tolerance test (ITT):

Time (mins)	0	20	30	60	90	120
Glucose (mmol/litre)	4	2	2	4.2	7.1	8.0
Cortisol (nmol/litre)	20	50	80	85	78	68
GH (mU/litre)	<0.5	0.6	0.6	<0.5	<0.5	<0.5
TSH (mU/litre)	3.1	14	30			
Prolactin (mU/litre)	699	1350	1010			

a)   What three endocrine anomalies does she have? (3 marks)

Select THREE answers only

☐ A Primary cortisol deficiency
☐ B Secondary cortisol deficiency
☐ C Growth hormone deficiency
☐ D Primary hyperprolactinaemia
☐ E Secondary hyperprolactinaemia
☐ F Primary hypothyroidism
☐ G Secondary hypothyroidism
☐ H Diabetes mellitus

b)   What treatments are required? (3 marks)

Select THREE answers only

☐ A Hydrocortisone
☐ B Fludrocortisone
☐ C Intranasal DDAVP
☐ D Thyroxine
☐ E Insulin
☐ F Bromocriptine
☐ G Growth hormone

QUESTION 5.11

A short 2-year-old boy has a long history of steatorrhoea and recurrent chest and skin infections.

Investigations

Hb:	10.1 g/dl
WBC:	3.5 × 10⁹/litre
Neutrophils:	17%
Platelets:	90 × 10⁹/litre
Faecal elastase:	150 (normal > 500)

Sweat test:
   Sodium: 21 mmol/litre
   Chloride: 23 mmol/litre
Femoral head X-rays: metaphyseal dysplasia

a) What is the diagnosis? (1 mark)

Select ONE answer only

- [ ] A Diamond–Blackfan syndrome
- [ ] B Cystic fibrosis
- [ ] C Schwachmann–Diamond syndrome
- [ ] D TAR syndrome
- [ ] E Fanconi anaemia

b) What medication should be used to treat the diarrhoea? (1 mark)

Select ONE answer only

- [ ] A Ursodeoxycholic acid
- [ ] B Loperamide
- [ ] C Kaolin
- [ ] D Sodium alginate
- [ ] E Pancreatic enzyme supplements

QUESTION 5.12

A baby is referred by the midwife with this nappy rash.

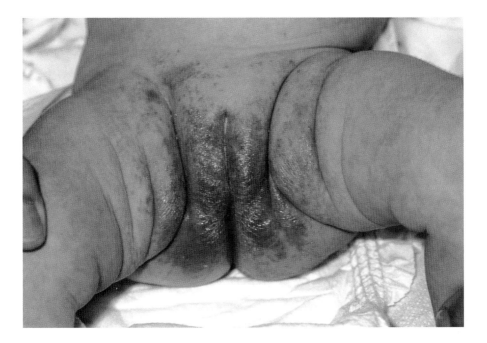

a)   What is most likely cause? (1 mark)

Select ONE answer only

- [ ] A *Candida* infection
- [ ] B Eczema
- [ ] C *Streptococcus* infection
- [ ] D *Staphylococcus* infection
- [ ] E Psoriasis

QUESTION 5.13

A full term baby boy was born weighing 3.95 kg. After some mild temperature fluctuation on the first day he was discharged home the following day. On the third day he is readmitted looking very ill and lethargic. A cannula is sited and blood obtained and a bolus of 20 ml/kg normal saline is given.

Investigations

Na: 132 mmol/litre
K: 4.7 mmol/litre
Bilirubin: 320 μmol/litre
Weight: 3.4 kg
Urine osmolarity: 88 mOsm/kg

a)   **What immediate management should be instituted? (1 mark)**

Select ONE answer only

☐ A   Electroencephalogram (EEG)
☐ B   Phototherapy
☐ C   Full septic screen including lumbar puncture and iv antibiotics
☐ D   Exchange transfusion
☐ E   Repeat fluid bolus

Following resuscitation more detailed studies are carried out:

Serum 17-hydroxyprogesterone: 2.6 nmol/litre (normal < 20 nmol/litre)
Plasma renin: high
Plasma aldosterone: low
Plasma ACTH: very high
Plasma cortisol: 96 nmol/litre
Urine Na: 90 mmol/litre
24 hour urine steroid profile:
    androgens: very low
    cortisol metabolites: very low

b) What is the most likely diagnosis? (1 mark)

Select ONE answer only

- ☐ A   Diabetes insipidus
- ☐ B   11-hydroxylase deficiency
- ☐ C   Renal tubular acidosis type I
- ☐ D   21-hydroxylase deficiency
- ☐ E   Congenital adrenal hypoplasia

c) What further treatment is required after initial resuscitation? (3 marks)

Select THREE answers only

- ☐ A   Sodium bicarbonate infusion
- ☐ B   Hydrocortisone
- ☐ C   Prednisolone
- ☐ D   Fludrocortisone
- ☐ E   Oral sodium supplements
- ☐ F   Acetazolamide
- ☐ G   Intranasal DDAVP
- ☐ H   Oral potassium supplements
- ☐ I   Chlorthiazide

QUESTION 5.14

An 11-month-old girl presents with a 3-day history of diarrhoea and vomiting. Over the past 24 hours she has become increasingly lethargic with occasional jerking movements of her lower limbs. On examination she looks 5–10% dehydrated, drowsy and difficult to rouse. Fontanelle feels full, but there is no neck stiffness and she is apyrexial with no rash and no lymphadenopathy.

Neurological examination reveals a full fontanelle, increased tone and brisk reflexes in her lower limbs with equivocal plantars. Fundi are normal.

Investigations

CSF:

RBC:	50/mm³
WBC:	3/mm³ lymphocytes

No organisms seen
Protein: 0.78 g/litre
Glucose: 2.2 mmol/litre

a) What one investigation will help make the diagnosis? (1 mark)

Select ONE answer only

- [ ] A   Plasma electrolytes
- [ ] B   CSF serology
- [ ] C   CSF culture
- [ ] D   CT brain scan
- [ ] E   EEG

b) What is the most likely diagnosis? (1 mark)

Select ONE answer only

- [ ] A   Sagittal sinus thrombosis
- [ ] B   Bacterial meningitis
- [ ] C   Viral encephalitis
- [ ] D   Intracranial tumour
- [ ] E   Benign raised intracranial pressure

QUESTION 5.15

Following a cricketing injury to his eye a 12-year-old boy presents to A&E with the following appearance.

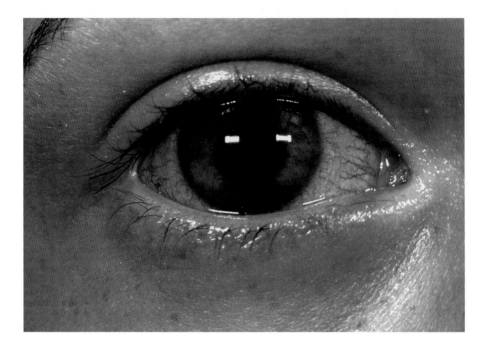

a) What is the diagnosis? (1 mark)

Select ONE answer only

☐ A Acute conjunctivitis
☐ B Acute episcleritis
☐ C Acute anterior uveitis
☐ D Hyphaema
☐ E Acute iritis

ANSWERS

PRACTICE EXAM 1 – ANSWERS

1.1 Answer

a) **A** – Barium meal and follow-through (1 mark)
   F – Colonoscopy and biopsy (2 marks)
b) **D** – Crohn's disease

Crohn's disease has increased in incidence to 5 per 100,000, equal to ulcerative colitis.

Whilst classical presentations are well known, several more unusual presentations are described. As it affects the entire GI tract, aphthous ulceration and cheilitis are important to note. The diagnosis has even been made after upper GI endoscopy revealing aphthous ulceration in the oesophagus. Anorexia nervosa is classically associated with a distorted body image, calorie counting, and other abnormal behaviour, which are uncharacteristic of inflammatory bowel disease.

An ESR or, more specifically, C-reactive protein with a barium meal and follow-through may give the diagnosis but the most useful diagnostic procedure is colonoscopy, with a biopsy to provide histological diagnosis.

Photo credit:

Dr P. Marazzi/Science Photo Library

References

Hyams JS. Crohn's disease in children. *Pediatr Clin N Am* 1996;**43**:255–77.
Walker-Smith JA. Clinical and diagnostic features of chronic inflammatory bowel
  disease in childhood. *Ballière's Clin Gastroenterol* 1994;**8**:65–82.

1.2 Answer

a) **A** – Blood culture
   C – Lumbar puncture for CSF glucose/protein/culture
   I – Serum calcium and magnesium levels
b) **C** – Inborn error of metabolism

This is a complex presentation with multiple possibilities. The question asks for immediate investigations, ie those that cannot be delayed prior to initial management. We know that the blood chemistry is normal and the glucose, whilst borderline, would not account for the seizures. With that in mind the clinical imperative would be to identify and manage correctable causes such as sepsis or calcium/magnesium deficiency.

Whilst a cranial ultrasound, congenital viral infection screen and urine toxicology may all be performed during the investigation of this child, they could all be done after initial management.

The timing of presentation is the key to this question as it relates to onset and restarting feeds. Opiate withdrawal, although possible, is generally either early in the case of maternal heroin withdrawal or late following exposure to methadone (which would probably be known about).

Inborn errors of metabolism generally present with vomiting, acidosis and circulatory disturbance followed by depressed consciousness and convulsions. Alternatively neurological features may dominate with hypotonia, lethargy, refusal to feed, progressing to unconsciousness and convulsions.

Reference

Hoffman GF. Selective screening for inborn errors of metabolism. *Eur J Pediatr* 1994;**153**(Suppl. 1):52–8.

1.3 Answer

a) **B** – Monospot test

There is an exudate over the tonsils and petechiae seen on the hard palate. This makes the most likely diagnosis glandular fever due to Epstein–Barr virus. The diagnosis can be confirmed using the Monospot or Paul Bunnell tests.

1.4 Answer

a) **D** – Right upper lobe consolidation with collapse
b) **E** – Specific serological testing
   G – Blood culture
c) **B** – Oral macrolide antibiotic

This is a typical history suggestive of an atypical pneumonia. Note also the anaemia, which would also be associated with a reticulocytosis suggestive of the cold agglutinins directed against red cells. Although these investigations would be helpful, they are not diagnostic tests. The budgerigar may be relevant because of the possibility of *Chlamydia psittaci*. However this causes bilateral patchy consolidation. The Heaf test at grade I is not suggestive of tuberculosis. The most likely organism is *Mycoplasma pneumoniae*.

In general it is not possible to differentiate the causative organism from the X-ray appearance (including differentiating viral from bacterial causes). *Mycoplasma pneumoniae* may produce a lobar pneumonia or a more atypical bilateral perihilar shadowing, with or without effusion.

A diagnostic pleural tap, which may be therapeutic, should be performed on any 'significant' pleural fluid to exclude an empyema, and cultured to aid diagnosis. Blood cultures should be performed in all unwell children with pneumonia – however, they are positive in less than 25%. Antibody titres, which often need to be measured in paired acute and convalescent samples, are the mainstay of diagnosis, but are often useful only retrospectively. The drug of choice for atypical pneumonias is a macrolide, which is equally as effective orally as intravenously.

Reference

Guidelines for the management of community acquired pneumonia in childhood. British Thoracic Society Standards of Care Committee. *Thorax* 2002;**57**(Suppl I).

1.5 Answer

a) 1. –E. Randomised control trial
    2. –A. Cross-sectional study
    3. –F. Clinical audit
    4. –C. Cohort study
    5. –C. Cohort study
    6. –D. Case control study
    7. –C. Cohort study

▪ *Cross-sectional studies*: a defined population is surveyed and their exposure and/or disease status determined at one point in time. This type of study allows prevalence, relative risk, and disease burden to be calculated. They are relatively quick and inexpensive to conduct. However, they are not suitable for the study of rare disease or diseases of short duration. As they provide a 'snap shot in time', causality and incidence cannot be shown.

■ *Geographical studies*: a defined population is examined using available statistics to look at the incidence of a disease and the incidence of exposure to a risk factor at a population level. This type of study is very easily and rapidly carried out at very low cost. It cannot however tell, at an individual level, whether those suffering from illness were exposed to the risk factor, and thus its main use is as an initial survey.

■ *Cohort studies*: a group of people is followed through time and the incidence in the exposed population is compared with the incidence in the unexposed population. Other measures that can be made in a cohort study include attributable risk and relative risk. A number of selection and recall biases are avoided by using this type of study. Large numbers of patients are required to study a rare disease – potentially they are long and expensive trials and maintaining follow-up is difficult.

■ *Case control studies*: compares the frequency of exposure to a risk factor in a representative group of cases, and a control group representative of the population from which the cases came. This is the best type of study to look at rare diseases. They are relatively cheap and require relatively few subjects. Rates of disease however cannot be determined, only compared, ie odds ratio. This type of study relies on recall and this may introduce a bias, validation is difficult and the selection of an appropriate control group is often difficult; it may also be difficult to show a temporal sequence.

■ *Randomised control trials*: an interventional type of trial, its main use is not in epidemiological study of disease aetiology but in the evaluation and comparison of treatment; however, by inference from the results, aetiological factors can be identified. The study, like a cohort study, is prospective but the investigator intervenes in one group and withholds intervention in the control. As intervention is needed, the volunteers must give informed consent. This consent may itself cause problems for the trial in that by informing a patient of their risk of a certain condition, they may then modify their lifestyle, and hence reduce their risk of getting the observed condition. This makes the statistical significance of an intervention more difficult to prove.

1.6 Answer

a) **D** – Erythema multiforme

Erythema multiforme is a cutaneous hypersensitivity reaction, which may follow infection or drugs but is often asymptomatic. The commonest cause of recurrent erythema multiforme is herpes simplex virus. Patients present with a sudden onset of symmetrical lesions with concentric colour changes (target lesions).

1.7 Answer

a) **G** – Bilateral moderate conductive hearing loss
b) **D** – Chronic suppurative otitis media

Measurements of the thresholds for air and bone conduction are usually obtained by pure tone audiometry. Stimuli of different frequencies ranging from 250 to 8000 Hz are emitted at different intensities above the threshold of normal hearing.

A sound made through a headphone of a standard audiometer will also be heard in the contralateral ear if the source in that ear is 50dB or greater. At this stage, masking of the non-test ear has to be undertaken.

For bone conduction testing, when a vibrator is placed on the skull, there is virtually no loss of sound heard in the non-test ear, thus masking should always be undertaken.

In this example there is a wide threshold between air conduction and bone conduction, an 'air–bone gap'. This implies the hearing loss is due to a malfunction of the conducting system of the external and middle ear, rather than a sensorineural mechanism.

Conductive deafness is the most common type of hearing loss in children. It may be due to chronic otitis media with effusion, acute otitis media or congenital abnormalities of the external or middle ear. In this case, the hearing loss is bilateral making chronic suppurative otitis media the most likely cause. Otosclerosis does cause bilateral conductive hearing loss but it is progressive and seen mainly in older patients.

Intermittent conductive deafness, provided speech and language are not delayed, is reviewed with audiograms and tympanometry and may resolve spontaneously. Persistent hearing loss from middle ear fluid is an indication for referral to an ENT surgeon for possible myringotomy/grommets or adenoidectomy.

1.8 Answer

a) **C** – X-linked dominant (2 marks)
    A – Autosomal dominant (1 mark)
b) **1.–F** – 50%
    2.–A – Zero
    3.–F – 50%
    4.–F – 50%

The inheritance pattern shown is most likely X-linked dominant. Although an autosomal dominant pattern is possible in V, there is no male-to-male transmission, making this unlikely. X-linked dominant conditions include X-linked hypophosphataemic rickets and ornithine transcarbamylase deficiency. Rett syndrome is thought to be X-linked dominant, although only females appear to be affected. It is thought that this condition is lethal *in utero* to males with no normal copy of the X chromosome.

In an X-linked dominant condition there is no carrier status and therefore the risk to the offspring of an unaffected individual is entirely due to new mutations. Male-to-male transmission does not occur.

Reference

Thompson, McInnes, Willard. 1982. *Thompson & Thompson, Genetics in Medicine*, 5th edn. W.B. Saunders.

1.9 Answer

a) A – Parvovirus B19

The red rash on this infant's face and arms is known as slapped cheek or fifth disease. Also called erythema infectiosum, this infectious disease is caused by parvovirus B19. It affects children between the ages of 2–14; outbreaks appear usually in the spring. Symptoms of a spreading red rash and a mild fever appear after an incubation period of between 4 and 14 days.

Photo credit:

Dr H.C. Robinson/Science Photo Library

1.10 Answer

a) **D** – Hypsarrhythmia
b) **D** – Tuberous sclerosis

EEG are common 'data interpretation questions'. They are not complicated and simply a matter of pattern recognition. You will need to know about seven 'patterns' as well as the normal trace. Here is a simple guide:

1. Read the question, noting the age and any drug treatment.

2. Check the time marker, usually at the top of the EEG in 1-second intervals. This allows calculation of the frequency of any complex.

3. Check the amplitude scale.

4. Check the montage (map). This is basically a pictorial representation of the sites between which a potential difference is being measured.

5. Now look at the traces: What is its nature – spike/sharp wave, slow wave, complex? Is it present in all channels (generalised) or only in one area (focal)?

6. Is there a pattern eg 3-per-second spike waves in absences, periodic complexes in subacute sclerosing panencephalitis, chaotic large voltage complexes in hypsarrhythmia, rolandic spikes?

In this case hypsarrhythmia is accompanied by developmental delay, and a CT with periventricular calcification, making tuberous sclerosis the most likely diagnosis.

1.11 Answer

a) **A** – Right axis deviation
   C – Right atrial enlargement
   H – Right ventricular hypertrophy
b) **B** – Ventricular septal defect
   F – Right ventricular outflow obstruction
c) **C** – Tetralogy of Fallot
d) **B** – Blalock–Taussig shunt

The ECG shows right axis deviation. There are prominent P waves in lead V1, which suggests right atrial enlargement. In the same lead the tall R wave and upright T waves are suggestive of right ventricular hypertrophy. Although these are often seen in tetralogy of Fallot, they may be absent and the ECG normal.

Cardiac catheter data are best interpreted by following saturations and then pressure measurements through each chamber in the anatomical sequence from systematic venous to systematic arterial.

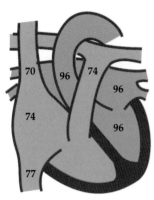

Normal Oxygen Saturations (%)   Normal Pressure Measurements (mmHg)

In tetralogy of Fallot the pulmonary stenosis results in a high right ventricular pressure and hence right ventricular hypertrophy. The large VSD and high right heart pressures cause a right-to-left shunt. The aorta is over the shunt as the VSD is high and thus there is also flow from the right ventricle directly into the aorta. The degree of pulmonary stenosis is variable (ranging from mild to atresia) so the clinical picture ranges in severity; the stenosis is often progressive.

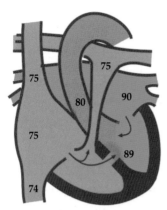

Oxygen Saturations in Tetralogy (%)

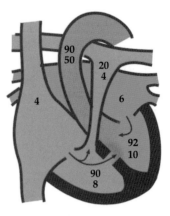

Pressure Measurements in Tetralogy (mmHg)

There is a step-up in oxygen saturation between right atrium and right ventricle implying a left-to-right shunt at a ventricular level. The pressure gradient between the right ventricle and pulmonary artery implies right ventricular outflow obstruction. These features, in addition to desaturation seen in the aorta (cyanosis) suggest the diagnosis of tetralogy of Fallot.

Symptomatic infants may require a Blalock–Taussig shunt, using a tube of Gortex to connect the subclavian artery to the pulmonary artery, which then provides a left-to-right shunt, replacing the duct as it closes.

Surgical correction is performed at 4–6 months under cardiopulmonary bypass, performed by opening the pulmonary stenosis (by patch enlargement where indicated) and closure of the VSD.

1.12 Answer

a) E – Osgood–Schlatter Disease

Osgood–Schlatter disease is a common cause of knee pain in the adolescent. During growth spurts, contraction of the strong quadriceps muscle is transmitted to the tibial tuberosity, which may result in a partial avulsion fracture through the ossification centre. Secondary bone formation may occur within the tendon near to its insertion causing the visible lump.

1.13 Answer

a) **A** – Hereditary spherocytosis
b) **C** – Osmotic fragility testing
c) **E** – Parvovirus B19

Unconjugated hyperbilirubinaemia with low haptoglobin suggests intravascular haemolysis, although hereditary spherocytosis, pyruvate kinase deficiency and glucose-6-phosphate dehydrogenase deficiency could all cause this, his father is also affected suggesting autosomal dominant transmission.

Hereditary spherocytosis is the most common of the inherited haemolytic states in which there is no abnormality of haemoglobin. The underlying defect is in the anchoring of the cell membrane to the cytoskeleton. The classic features are a congenital (autosomal dominant, but 25% are new mutations) haemolytic process associated with splenomegaly and spherical red cells. Pigment gallstones usually develop late in childhood and aplastic crises associated with parvovirus are serious complications. Spherocytes seen on blood film are not diagnostic as they may occur in other conditions; the diagnostic test demonstrates the osmotic fragility of cells. Splenectomy may be required to reduce haemolysis, but is deferred until the patient is 6 years of age.

1.14 Answer

a) 1.–E
   2.–C
   3.–G
   4.–F
   5.–B

	Calcium	Phosphate	ALP	Parathyroid	25 (OH) Vit D
1° Hyperparathyroidism	High	Low	Normal/high	High	Normal
2° Hyperparathyroidism	Normal/low	High	High	High	Normal
X-linked hypophosphataemic rickets	Normal	Very low	High	Normal	Normal/low
Vitamin D deficiency	Low/ normal	Low/normal	High	High	Low
Vitamin D dependent rickets	Low	Low/normal	High	High	Normal

1.15 Answer

a) **C** – Left 4th cranial nerve palsy

The photograph shows a divergent squint resulting from a congenital IV cranial nerve palsy. The resulting weakness in the superior oblique muscle causes the eye to be diverted down and outwards due to the unopposed action of the other muscles supplied by the abducens (VI) and oculomotor (III) nerves.

Photo credit:

Dr P. Marazzi/Science Photo Library

PRACTICE EXAM 2 – ANSWERS

2.1 Answer

a) **D** – Severe combined immune deficiency
b) **D** – *Pneumocystis jiroveci* (previously known as *Pneumocystis carinii*)
c) **E** – Intravenous co-trimoxazole

This is a familial immune deficiency with early onset. Early death in a first-degree relative should arouse suspicion of recessively inherited disorder. There is panhypogammaglobulinaemia with low normal white count. Human immune deficiency virus causes a hypergammaglobulinaemia and lymphadenopathy, which are absent. There is no full differential white count given but it can be calculated that the absolute eosinophil count is 1.7, giving a combined neutrophil and lymphocyte count of 3.3, which is low.

Bruton's agammaglobulinaemia is X-linked and, as a previous affected sibling was female, this is unlikely. Agammaglobulinaemia usually presents at 4–6 months when maternally transferred antibodies are exhausted. The presence of diarrhoea from birth suggests the presence of a cellular deficiency in addition to humoral deficiency.

Wiskott–Aldrich syndrome is a possibility but usually is associated with thrombocytopenia, increased IgA, normal IgG and half-normal IgM levels. Severe combined immune deficiency (SCID) has many familial forms in both autosomal and sex-linked recessive forms. The rash may be chronic candida.

Functional antibodies such as isohaemagglutinins will be absent and there will be absent sensitivity to candida skin testing. Chronic rotavirus carriage is common.

Management is supportive until a matched bone marrow donor becomes available. Any blood products required must be irradiated to prevent a graft versus host reaction.

2.2 Answer

a) **F** – Renal vein thrombosis
b) **D** – Abdominal ultrasound scan
c) **A** – Hypernatraemia
   D – Intracranial haemorrhage
   G – Hypertension

The age of the child, preceding diarrhoea and palpable kidney make the diagnosis likely. Although the clinical presentation would fit with a GI problem (intussusception, malrotation, volvulus), the presence of haematuria, uraemia and thrombocytopenia make renal vein thrombosis the most likely diagnosis.

One-third of all cases of renal vein thrombosis are detected in the first week of life. Severity varies from grave bilateral involvement to focal involvement of one kidney. Asphyxia, prematurity, dehydration, sepsis and maternal diabetes are possible predisposing factors. In severe cases, peritoneal dialysis and intensive care on a paediatric nephrology unit is indicated. Careful follow-up is required, as the affected kidney may cause severe hypertension via a renin-mediated pathway and should, in that case, be removed.

Reference

Andrew M, Booker LA. 1996. Hemostatic complications in renal disorders of the young. *Pediatr Nephrol* **10**:88–99.

2.3 Answer

a) **E** – Ulcerative colitis

The X-ray shows a lead pipe appearance of the transverse and descending colon with loss of normal anatomical features. In view of the confluent nature of the lesion and the part of the bowel affected, the most likely diagnosis is ulcerative colitis.

2.4 Answer

a) **E** – Ketotic hypoglycaemia
b) **A** – Provocation fast

In nesidioblastosis there is a pancreatic anomaly resulting in autonomous insulin secretion not controlled by plasma glucose levels. It usually presents between infancy and 18 months of life with hypoglycaemia, and newborns are often macrosomic.

Medium chain acyl-Co-A dehydrogenase (MCAD) deficiency is the commonest fatty acid oxidation disorder. Hypoglycaemia is usually precipitated by prolonged fasts of 12–16 hours. Episodes often progress to coma and cardiorespiratory collapse. Ketones are characteristically low in the presence of hypoglycaemia.

Children with type I glycogen storage disease become very tolerant to hypoglycaemia and do not have classical symptoms of hypoglycaemia. Untreated they have severe developmental delay.

Glycogen synthetase deficiency is rare. Hypoglycaemia and elevated ketones occur on fasting; however, following a meal hyperglycaemia occurs.

Ketotic hypoglycaemia is the most common cause of hypoglycaemia and presents usually between 1 and 5 years of age. Affected children (usually boys, M:F 2:1) are small and thin. The basic biochemical defect is unknown but hepatic glycogen is known to be depleted and it is postulated that there is a failure in mobilisation of amino acids from muscle for gluconeogenesis in starvation. Owing to accelerated starvation, free fatty acid oxidation is increased giving the disorder its name.

The diagnosis is established by excluding metabolic errors and hormone deficiencies. Either with a carefully supervised fast or prior to a spontaneous episode of hypoglycaemia, urine will become ketotic before hypoglycaemia occurs and serial blood glucose measurements should demonstrate hypoglycaemia within 8–16 hours. Simultaneous measurements should be as follows:

Insulin: low
GH: elevated
Cortisol: elevated
Thyroxine: normal

Free fatty acid: elevated

Betahydroxybutyrate: elevated

Ketones: elevated

Amino acids: decreased alanine (used for gluconeogenesis)

2.5 Answer

a) **1.–E** – The 'unbearable' situation
  2.–D – The 'no purpose' situation
  3.–B – The 'permanent vegetative' state
  4.–D – The 'no purpose' situation
  5.–C – The 'no chance' situation

- *The 'brain dead' child*: irreversible cessation of all functions of the entire brain or irreversible cessation of all functions of the entire brain including the brain stem. Of note is the criterion of brain death and its testing is not appropriate in neonates owing to immaturity of brain responses.

- *The 'permanent vegetative' state*: the child who develops a permanent vegetative state following insults, such as trauma or hypoxia, is reliant on others for all care and does not react or relate with the outside world. This state is deemed persistent if it lasts for 4 weeks or more, and permanent if it is predicted that awareness will not recover.

- *The 'no chance' situation*: the child has such severe disease that life-sustaining treatment simply delays death without alleviation of suffering.

- *The 'no purpose' situation*: although the child may be able to survive with treatment, the degree of mental or physical impairment would be so great that it is unreasonable to expect the child to bear it.

- *The unbearable situation*: the child and/or family feel that, in the face of progressive and irreversible illness, further treatment is more than can be borne. They wish to have a particular treatment withdrawn or to refuse further treatment irrespective of the medical opinion that it may be of some benefit.

Reference

RCPCH. 2004. *Withholding and withdrawing life saving treatment in children*, 2nd edn. London: Royal College of Paediatrics and Child Health.

2.6 Answer

a) **E** – Scarlet fever

Scarlet fever (or scarlatina) is a childhood disease caused by group A beta haemolytic *Streptococcus*. It is spread by droplets of fluid, coughed, sneezed or breathed into the air. Symptoms occur 2–4 days after exposure and include fever, sore throat and a widespread red rash affecting the torso, limbs and tongue. The rash is caused by an exotoxin.

Photo credit:

Biophoto Associates/Science Photo Library

2.7 Answer

a) **D** – 3-per-second spike and wave activity
b) **C** – Hyperventilation
c) **A** – None

In childhood absence epilepsy, the age of onset is 3–13 years. Neurological examination is normal. Although intelligence is normal, development may be delayed if absences are very frequent. Seizures are typical absences (simple or complex) at onset, possibly followed by generalised tonic clonic seizures.

The EEG has a normal background, with ictal episodes of synchronous, symmetrical spike waves, usually at 3 Hz spontaneously and/or activated by hyperventilation.

If these criteria are satisfied, further neuroimaging is not necessary prior to treatment.

2.8 Answer

a) **B** – Mildly delayed gross motor development
  D – Normal fine motor development
  H – Mildly delayed speech and language development
b) **A** – Acquired immunodeficiency syndrome (AIDS)

Maternofetal transmission is responsible for 80% of paediatric HIV infection in the UK. With routine screening of blood products, the number of children infected through transfusion of blood or blood products has been minimised.

Without preventative strategies the vertical transmission rate is 30%. Each intervention halves the rate of transmission: maternal retroviral use, caesarean birth, retrovirals to the neonate, no breast feeding, which all reduce the transmission rate in the UK to 1–2%.

Of those children presenting, 75% have non-specific problems such as failure to thrive, recurrent bacterial infections, chronic diarrhoea, or skin infections. There may also be hepatosplenomegaly and lymphadenopathy. Polyclonal hypergammaglobulinaemia is sensitive and specific as early as 3 months.

Neurodevelopmental findings include developmental delay, regression of developmental milestones, acquired microcephaly and gait abnormalities.

2.9 Answer

a) **E** – Erythema chronicum migrans

The rash is associated with Lyme disease; an asymmetrical arthritis, which involves large joints, was first described in Connecticut in 1972. This form of arthritis follows 1–24 weeks after the rash and is due to *Borrelia burgdorferi*. The infection is transmitted by a tick of the genus *Ixodes*.

Photo credit:

John Radcliffe Hospital/Science Photo Library

2.10 Answer

a) **A.** Neonatal RS progression
   C. Prolonged PR interval
   H. Superior axis
b) **C.** Atrioventricular septal defect (probably in a baby with Down syndrome)

2.11 Answer

a) **C** – Partially treated bacterial meningitis.

Typical findings in the CSF after the first year of life are as follows:

	Normal	**Bacterial**	**Viral**
Appearance	Clear	Cloudy	Clear
Cells/mm³	0–5	100–100,000	10–1000
	Lymphocytes	neutrophils	lymphocytes
Glucose	> 50% blood	< 50% blood	50% blood
Protein g/l	0.2–0.5	1–5	0.5–2

(NB. Mumps meningitis can cause a low glucose.)

2.12 Answer

a) **A** – Quinsy

The photo shows a close-up of the mouth with a left-sided pus-filled abscess (centre right of picture) around the base of a tonsil in quinsy. This peritonsillar abscess is usually a complication of tonsillitis. Symptoms include fever, pain on swallowing or opening the mouth, headache and swollen lymph nodes in the neck. Antibiotic drugs may clear the infection, but often surgical drainage of the abscess is necessary, followed by removal of the tonsils.

Photo credit:

Dr P. Marazzi/Science Photo Library

2.13 Answer

a) 1. **E** – Increase the I:E ratio
    2. **G** – Increase the rate
    3. **A** – Increase the peak inspiratory pressure (PIP)
    4. **C** – Increase the positive end expiratory pressure (PEEP)
    5. **D** – Decrease the positive end expiratory pressure (PEEP)

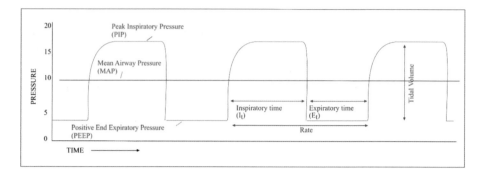

Physiologically, oxygenation is dependent on the mean airway pressure (the area under the curve). To increase it, the peak inspiratory pressure or the positive end expiratory pressure can be increased or the I time prolonged (increased I:E ratio).

Carbon dioxide elimination is dependent on minute ventilation, which is the tidal volume multiplied by the ventilation rate. The tidal volume is directly proportional to the tidal pressure (if ventilating on the correct part of the compliance curve). Thus to increase carbon dioxide elimination, the tidal pressure can be increased (increase peak inspiratory pressure or reduce the positive end expiratory pressure) or increase the rate.

2.14 Answer

a) **F** – Right baggy collecting system
    H – Reduced right differential function
b) **E** – Furosemide iv

MAG3 is a dynamic renal imaging technique. The basic scan as shown involves examining the uptake of tracer by the functioning kidney and then its passage through the nephrons, to the collecting system and into the urine. In renal artery stenosis the gradient of the affected kidney is much shallower.

In this scan the right kidney takes up much less tracer than the left (highest point on the graph); therefore there is reduced differential function on that side. Initially it appears that there is renal outflow obstruction; however, after the administration of furosemide (at point 'A'), the tracer passes rapidly out of the kidney showing the collecting system to be baggy rather than truly obstructed.

A further part of the study that can be carried out (not shown in this example) is indirect micturating cystography. Once all the tracer has passed into the bladder the child is asked to pass urine whilst the camera is trained on the lower ends of the ureters. If there is a spike of activity during micturition this demonstrates vesicoureteric reflux, making a micturating cystourogram and hence bladder catheterisation unnecessary.

2.15 Answer

a) **A** – Microcytosis
   C – Anisocytosis
   D – Poikilocytosis
   K – Pencil cells
b) **D** – Iron deficiency anaemia

This is a light micrograph of a blood smear in a patient suffering from iron deficiency anaemia. Cells appear poorly stained (hypochromasia), irregularly shaped (poikilocytosis) and smaller than normal (microcytosis) with varying sizes (anisocytosis).

Photo credit:

Dr E. Walker/Science Photo Library

PRACTICE EXAM 3 – ANSWERS

3.1 Answer

a) **C** – Acute lymphoblastic leukaemia
b) **A** – Full blood count
   E – Bone marrow aspirate

This is a multisystem disease with several key features in the history:

- Bleeding disorder – unexplained bruise on thigh

- Fever and sore throat

- Spinal cord lesion in the lumbar region

- Possible meningeal irritation – stiff neck and back

Acute lymphoblastic leukaemia with meningeal infiltration is the most likely diagnosis.

Acute leukaemia is the commonest malignancy of childhood, the leukaemias together account for 30% of childhood cancers. About 70% are acute lymphoblastic (ALL), 20% acute myeloblastic (AML) or variants.

Prognosis

- ALL better than AML

- Common and T cell better than B cell

- High WBC at presentation > 60,000 carries poor prognosis

- Age at presentation < 1 year or > 14 years poor prognosis

- Presence of CNS involvement at diagnosis is an unfavourable feature

- Prognosis is better if remission achieved within 14 days of induction.

Photo credit:

Astrid & Hanns-Frieder Michler/Science Photo Library

3.2 Answer

a) **A** – Distal intestinal obstruction syndrome
   E – Appendix abscess
   F – Intussusception
b) **C** – Contrast enema

Distal intestinal obstruction syndrome (previously known as meconium ileus equivalent) can produce intestinal obstruction in cystic fibrosis at any age. Prior to complete obstruction, increasing pancreatic enzyme supplements and oral fluid intake may be all that is required. In more severe cases oral gastrograffin may relieve obstruction. Once the obstruction is complete (as suggested by this history), a gastrograffin enema, provided the patient is stable with no signs of perforation or dehydration, can be diagnostic and therapeutic.

Where presumptive cases of distal intestinal obstruction syndrome fail to respond to the above measures, intussusception and appendix abscess must be considered.

3.3 Answer

a) **D** – Right sided congenital diaphragmatic hernia

3.4 Answer

a) **C** – Guillain–Barré syndrome
b) **E** – Nerve conduction studies and **C**. Lumbar puncture also acceptable
c) **A** – Spirometry

There are several key features in the history:

■ The past history of meningitis is irrelevant

■ Expressionless face is a clue to the facial weakness.

This child had a 3-day history of limb weakness, facial weakness and double vision with absent peripheral reflexes. The imminent danger is of respiratory muscle involvement with consequent respiratory failure.

Lumbar puncture may show cyto-albumin dissociation (high albumin with normal cell count); nerve conduction studies are of assistance in making the diagnosis at an early stage. The differential diagnosis would be myasthenia gravis.

3.5 Answer

a) **E** – Complete heart block
b) **B** – Systemic lupus erythematosus

The heart rate shown on this ECG is around 75 bpm. Whilst normal in an older child or adult this is significantly low for a neonate. The rhythm strip shows that there is complete dissociation between the P waves and the QRS complexes. There is an association with maternal systemic lupus erythematosus owing to damage of the fetal conduction system by maternal auto-antibodies (anti-Ro/anti-La). Other rare associations include rheumatoid arthritis and dermatomyositis.

Symptomatic neonates (hydrops/congestive cardiac failure) may require cardiac pacing.

3.6 Answer

a) **E** – Arrange an abdominal ultrasound scan.

The photo shows a purpuric rash on the lower limbs and some inflammation of the ankles. This is due to Henoch–Schönlein purpura (HSP). Although the abdominal pain may result from mesenteric vasculitis, patients with HSP are at increased risk of developing intussusception. An abdominal ultrasound scan will help to exclude this. Once intussusception has been excluded, the abdominal pain may be managed by simple analgesics. Refractory cases may benefit from a short course of oral steroids.

3.7 Answer

a) **1. B** – < 1%
    2. B – < 1%
    3. F – 50%
    4. F – 50%

The photograph shows a child with short limbs and marked lumbar lordosis due to achondroplasia. The inheritance pattern of achondroplasia is autosomal dominant; however, four-fifths of cases are new mutations, born to unaffected patients. Although neither parent is affected, the risk of having another affected child is above that for the general population (1 in 50,000), as one parent may exhibit gonadal mosaicism.

3.8 Answer

a) **C** – Thyroid function tests
   E – Chromosomes
b) **B** – Primary hypothyroidism

Delayed bone age and declining height velocity are firm reasons to investigate this girl's short stature. Turner's syndrome and hypothyroidism should be considered in any teenage girl who presents in this way, even if the clinical features are not obvious.

In a standard insulin tolerance test there should be an appropriate hypoglycaemia, GH should rise to exceed 12.5, cortisol should double its base level and FSH/LH should rise in parallel to GnRH challenge.

In this example, the GH response is borderline low but the most striking abnormality is the very high baseline TSH, which is unresponsive to TRH, implying this is primary organ-associated hypothyroidism.

Thyroxine replacement therapy should be commenced with great care because of side effects in the cardiovascular system. Progress should be monitored symptomatically and by the TSH level. Parents should be warned that a previous inactive docile child will become more energetic and that school performance may suffer until stabilisation is attained.

3.9 Answer

a) **A.** Varicella zoster

The small white lesions on the back of an 11-year-old boy's mouth are due to chickenpox. Two weeks after initial infection a red, pruritic vesicular eruption occurs on the trunk, upper arms and legs, and inside the mouth and trachea causing a dry cough. This is accompanied by fever.

Photo credit:

Dr P. Marazzi/Science Photo Library

3.10 Answer

a) **E** – Kawasaki's disease
b) **B** – Serological testing
   D – Throat swab
   E – ASO titre
c) **A** – Immunoglobulin i.v.

Diagnostic criteria

■ Fever > 5 days unresponsive to antibiotics, and at least four of the five following physical findings with no other more reasonable explanation for the observed clinical findings:

   – bilateral conjunctival injection

   – oral mucosal changes (erythema of lips or oropharynx, strawberry tongue, or drying or fissuring of the lips)

   – peripheral extremity changes (oedema, erythema, or generalised or desquamation)

   – rash

   – cervical lymphadenopathy > 1.5 cm in diameter

However, atypical cases with shorter duration of fever are increasingly being recognised and there is an association with the formation of a granuloma at the site of previous BCG vaccination. In this case the raised platelet count helps make Kawasaki's disease stand out as the most likely from the list of disorders causing desquamation. There are no diagnostic tests, and waiting for a further rise in platelet count could be dangerous. Serology may rule out measles; ASOT and throat swab help to rule out scarlet fever.

These tests should not delay the administration of immunoglobulin. The child should also be started on aspirin. Acute and convalescent echocardiograms should be arranged to look for coronary artery aneurysms.

Reference

Center for Disease Control, 1980. Kawasaki disease – New York. *Mortal Morbid Wkly Rep* **29**:61–63.

3.11 Answer

a) **B** – Encephalitis
b) **E** – Herpes simplex virus

EEG are common 'data interpretation questions'. For a general approach see the answer to question 1.10. In this case there are focal areas of slow waves suggesting a focal encephalitis.

3.12 Answer

a) **A** – Congenital glaucoma

This is a close-up of the eyes of a child suffering from congenital glaucoma. Both eyes have fluid leaking from the eyeball into the gap between the lens and the cornea, seen as a slight clearing around each pupil. The right eye is also slightly enlarged. Congenital glaucoma is due to a structural abnormality in the drainage angles of the eyes. Normal fluid drainage is impaired and pressure builds up, damaging the eye's internal structures. The eyeball can become hard and painful when the condition develops acutely. Treatments include diuretic drugs or drainage surgery.

Photo credit:

Sue Ford/Science Photo Library

3.13 Answer

a) **A** – Blood film
   C – Bone marrow aspiration
   G – Reticulocyte count
b) **E** – Diamond–Blackfan syndrome

The baby's anaemia is not due to Rhesus (negative DAT) or ABO incompatibility (baby is blood group O). The white count and platelets are normal. Diamond–Blackfan syndrome (pure red cell aplasia) usually presents with profound anaemia by 2–6 months. The most important diagnostic feature is the absence of red cell precursors in blood and bone marrow. Erythropoietin levels are high.

Treatment is supportive with transfusions and steroids. A few cases remit spontaneously, otherwise death occurs in the second decade without bone marrow transplantation.

3.14 Answer

a) 1. **I** – Knows first name
2. **D** – Builds a tower of 8 bricks
3. **G** – Stands on one foot for 6 seconds
4. **F** – Able to undress
5. **H** – Draws a recognisable man
6. **B** – Rides a tricycle
7. **C** – Uses a knife and fork at the table
8. **A** – Cuts a strip off the edge of a square of paper
9. **E** – Runs and kicks a ball

Developmental assessment questions are not uncommon in the MRCPCH. It is important to read the question structure as some refer to the 'normal' age at a milestone gained and some refer to the age at which not having achieved a milestone is 'abnormal'. This question uses milestones from the Griffiths Mental Development Scales, which are the most commonly used in paediatric practice.

One approach to this question if you were unfamiliar with the milestones given would be to look at each milestone and decide whether it is locomotor, personal and social, or eye–hand coordination. Each category would then have three milestones, which can then be arranged into the apparent order of complexity and the answer deduced in that way.

3.15 Answer

a) **C** – Reassure parents, and discharge with antipyretics

The photo shows the recovery phase of acute secretory otitis media due to the presence of bubbles. There is some minor tympanosclerosis. The majority of otitis media is viral in origin; antibiotics are only indicated if the child is systemically unwell from a presumed bacterial infection.

Photo credit:

Professor Tony Wright, Institute Of Laryngology & Otology/Science Photo Library

PRACTICE EXAM 4 – ANSWERS

4.1 Answer

a) **D** – Hirschsprung's disease
b) **A** – Congenital hypothyroidism

Congenital hypothyroidism has an incidence of 1 in 3000, three times as common in girls as in boys. Thyroid hormone is known to cross the placenta and hence newborns have some initial sparing of features. Hirschsprung's is a related condition and should be confirmed with a rectal biopsy.

The clinical features of congenital hypothyroidsm are shown below (adapted from Robertson NRC. *A Textbook of Neonatology*. Churchill Livingstone). Note that this child was born abroad and may have missed the normal neonatal blood spot screening.

Features which may be present at birth:

- Postmature, large size

- Wide posterior fontanelle

- Umbilical hernia

- Goitre

Early signs, < 4 weeks

- Placid, 'good', sleeps a lot

- Poor feeder

- Constipation, abdominal distension

- Mottled, cold

- Oedema

- Prolonged jaundice

Late signs

- Cretinous appearance

- Big tongue

- Hoarse cry

- Dry skin and hair

- Slow responses

- Retarded growth and development.

Several other neurological deficits have been described including deafness, ataxia, attention deficit disorder, abnormal muscle tone and speech defects.

Photo credit:

Biophoto Associates/Science Photo Library

4.2 Answer

a) **1. A** – Pulmonary hypertension
   2. C – Atrial fibrillation
   3. E – Pulmonary embolism

A loud second heart sound (presumed P2) accompanied by a diastolic murmur signifies pulmonary hypertension with functional valvular incompetence. The irregular pulse signifies atrial fibrillation, which is then further complicated by a pulmonary embolism, which causes the chest pain and blood-stained sputum. Patch detachment following VSD repair is an early complication.

4.3 Answer

a) **E** – Foreign body left main bronchus

A foreign body aspirated into the bronchus may cause a complete obstruction resulting in a collapsed lung. A partial obstruction, however, may result in air trapping (ball valve effect) and hence over inflation of the affected lung. In a cooperative child this effect can be accentuated using paired inspiratory and expiratory chest X-rays.

4.4 Answer

a)   **D** – X-linked recessive
b) **1. A** – Zero
   2. E – 25%

4.5 Answer

a) **B** – Subacute sclerosing panencephalitis
b) **B** – CSF serology

Key points

- Cerebral changes many years after primary infection

- Insidious deterioration of higher cerebral function

- Elevated measles CSF antibody titre

- Periodic complexes on EEG.

This illness is rarely seen following the introduction of measles vaccine. School failure is often the first sign of a subtle deterioration in higher cerebral function. Generalised myoclonic jerks at regular intervals are characteristic. The EEG typically shows repeated bursts of generalised high-voltage slow wave complexes. In this girl the electromyographic record shows associated myoclonus.

4.6 Answer

a) **B** – Measles

The photos show the morbilliform rash and Koplik's spots in the mouth of a child suffering from measles. Koplik's spots are red with white centres and are a frequent symptom in this highly infectious viral disease that mainly affects children. Symptoms of cold and fever develop after an incubation period of 8–15 days. On the days 3–5 the characteristic blotchy rash develops, which progresses from the head down the body and persists for 3–5 days. The patient remains infectious throughout this period. In most cases the symptoms subside, but the child may be susceptible to pneumonia and infections of the middle ear. Complete recovery may take 2–4 weeks. Vaccination provides effective immunity against the disease.

Photo credit:

CNRI. Dr P. Marazzi Science Photo Library

4.7 Answer

a) **J** – Bilateral severe sensorineural hearing loss
b) **C** – *Streptococcus pneumoniae*

Following the introduction of HiB vaccination *H. influenzae* is now rarely seen. Pneumococcal meningitis is the most likely to cause such severe deafness. Note also that:

- Only unmasked bone conduction is obtained in severe binaural disease.

- The air–bone gap at 250 and 500 Hz is false at levels around 50 dBHL; bone conduction thresholds are felt through vibration ('vibration thresholds').

- Bone conduction thresholds are only measurable down to 60 dBHL and the presence of a false air–bone gap therefore appears in severe or profound loss.

4.8 Answer

a) **B** – Ventricular septal defect with left-to-right shunting
   E – Patent ductus arteriosus with right-to-left shunting
   G – Coarctation of the aorta
b) **D** – Intravenous prostaglandin

A general approach and normal values for cardiac catheterisation are given in the answer to question 1.11. When each chamber is worked through sequentially as previously outlined, there is a significant step-up in saturation at the right ventricular level indicating a ventricular septal defect with left-to-right shunt. The step-down at the aortic level confirms right-to-left shunting through a patent ductus arteriosus.

The history describes a preductal (infantile) coarctation, in which persistence of the ductus arteriosus is a common feature. The descending aorta receives most of its blood supply from the main pulmonary artery via the ductus arteriosus, while the left ventricle continues to supply the first two or three aortic branches. The pulmonary hypertension initially accompanies a high pulmonary blood flow, but may later reflect increasing pulmonary resistance.

In preductal coarctation, congestive cardiac failure is often precipitated in the earliest days or weeks of life. If possible, the preductal segment is excised and either end-to-end anastomosis or subclavian patch repair performed, followed by surgical closure of the ductus arteriosus.

4.9 Answer

a) A – Neurofibromatosis type I
    E – McCune–Albright syndrome
    H – Tuberous sclerosis
    L – Fanconi's anaemia

Café au lait (CAL) spots are hyperpigmented lesions. The size and number of CAL skin lesions vary greatly, and they are the earliest manifestations of neurofibromatosis type I. They may also occur sporadically in McCune–Albright syndrome, tuberous sclerosis, Fanconi's anaemia and occasionally in neurofibromatosis type II.

Photo credit:

Science Photo Library

4.10 Answer

a) A – Epstein–Barr virus
b) C – Monospot test

Clinical presentation of infectious mononucleosis is variable:

General features:

■ Fever, lymphadenopathy, pharyngitis, splenomegaly (50%)

■ Mild hepatomegaly, jaundice

Cardiac: Myocarditis, arrhythmias

Neurological: Aseptic meningitis, cranial nerve palsies, transverse myelitis

Haematological:

■ Atypical monocytes 5–50% total white count, actually transformed T cells

■ Autoimmune haemolytic anaemia with cold agglutinins

■ Thrombocytopenia

Whilst *Mycoplasma* may produce a similar clinical picture, the atypical cells seen on blood film makes infectious mononucleosis the most likely diagnosis.

Investigations

The heterophile antibody test is occasionally negative in early stages of infectious mononucleosis and may also give false positive results. Specific IgM antibody to EBV indicates a very recent or current infection.

4.11 Answer

a) **C** – Juvenile dermatomyositis
b) **F** – Muscle biopsy
   H – EMG
c) **B** – Prednisolone 1–2 mg/kg/day

Key points

- Inflammation of smooth muscle with typical cutaneous heliotrope rash

- Occlusive vasculitis

- Raised transaminases, CK

This is a multisystem disease characterised by inflammation of striated muscle, and typical cutaneous lesions. In muscle there is patchy degeneration, atrophy and regeneration. The most prominent lesion is an occlusive vasculitis. Myositis is predominant in proximal muscles.

The upper eyelids have a pathognomonic violaceous discolouration (heliotrope rash). Calcium may be deposited in affected subcutaneous tissues.

Of those children diagnosed with juvenile dermatomyositis 50–60% will have a positive ANA. The EMG of affected muscles is abnormal.

Severe involvement of the palatorespiratory muscles may affect breathing, and in these children intubation and ventilation may be necessary. Physiotherapy to avoid contractures as well as steroid therapy are the recommended treatments.

4.12 Answer

a) **B** – Primary herpes gingivostomatitis

Generally caused by herpes simplex type I virus, gingivostomatitis is a common childhood primary manifestation. After a prodromal illness the child develops painful ulcerating lesions in the mouth associated with high pyrexia and, commonly, refusal to drink. Admission to hospital for nasogastric hydration may be required.

4.13 Answer

a) **A** – Coeliac disease
b) **C** – Upper GI endoscopy and biopsy

It is important not to be distracted by issues such as congenital heart disease or drug therapies. Although congenital heart disease is responsible for poor growth in some circumstances, contained within this question is the classical description of a child presenting with coeliac disease. Note also the timing of failure to thrive occurring after early weaning due to the coeliac disease.

Coeliac disease is a gluten-induced enteropathy requiring characteristic histological findings to confirm the diagnosis. Increasing use is made of anti-gliadin and endomysial antibodies although it must be remembered to also send a total IgA at the same time (IgA deficiency is often associated and will give a false negative result). Transient gluten intolerance is more common before the age of 1 and therefore a rechallenge with gluten should be carried out after a year on a gluten-free diet.

4.14 Answer

a) **A** – Reversible obstructive airways disease
   G – Increased residual volume

Obstructive lung disease (reduced FEV_1/FVC) is often defined as reversible if, following administration of a bronchodilator, there is a 15% improvement in FEV_1. Airways disease accelerates the increase in residual volume. Any airways narrowing or loss of recoil, allowing dynamic compression, facilitates air trapping within the lungs and hence increased residual volume is also characteristic of obstructive airways disease.

The total lung capacity depends on the balance of the ability of the respiratory muscles to expand the chest and the tendency of the lungs and chest wall to recoil inwards towards their resting position. The increase in lung disease is due primarily to the loss of elastic recoil, often related to localised damage with cysts or bullae.

4.15 Answer

a) **D** – EEC syndrome

The feet show ectrodactyly, absence of all or part of one or more digits. Ectrodactyly is one condition of the EEC syndrome, which is a form of ectodermal dysplasia. EEC stands for ectrodactyly, ectodermal dysplasia and clefting syndrome. Although it is an inherited developmental disorder, there can be considerable variation in the level of expression between affected members of the same family. The gene responsible for EEC syndrome is P63. Other characteristics of ectodermal dysplasias are missing or malformed teeth, abnormality of hair growth and irregular skin pigmentation.

Photo credit:

Science Photo Library

PRACTICE EXAM 5 – ANSWERS

5.1 Answer

a) **C** – Right middle lobe consolidation
b) **A** – Immunoglobulins
   F – Sweat test
   H – Nasal brushings
c) **B** – Primary ciliary dyskinesia

All the information in the question is relevant – do not miss points. It is important to note the serous otitis media, thriving child and stomach bubble on the right.

A number of conditions with abnormalities of ciliary function are now recognised. Kartagener's syndrome classically implies situs inversus, sinusitis and bronchiectasis. It is inherited in an autosomal recessive manner. Although classically the apex of the heart would be on the right, there is a variant of situs inversus with levocardia where the apex of the heart is on the left. This has no correlation with the internal arrangement of the heart (which may still be reversed). Only 50% of cases of primary ciliary dyskinesia have situs inversus.

As the condition is present from birth, these patients have a history of respiratory distress at birth. Later chronic upper and lower respiratory tract disease is almost universal. There is a strong correlation with chronic suppurative otitis media and conductive hearing loss.

Diagnosis requires nasal brushings and immediate motility studies by photometric means. Electron microscopy shows a wide variety of structural defects including defective dynein arms or missing spokes.

As the problem is a structural one it is irreversible and so management involves antibiotics, physiotherapy, with the objective of preventing or delaying bronchiectasis, and ENT intervention as required. Many males are infertile, so appropriate sperm mobility tests and counselling should be carried out.

Reference

Corbeel L *et al*. 1981. Ultrastructural abnormalities of bronchial cilia in children with recurrent airway infection and bronchiectasis. *Arch Dis Child* **56**:929–33.

5.2 Answer

a) **D** – X-linked recessive (autosomal recessive is possible but not the most likely)
b) **B** – Autosomal recessive
c) **E** – > 95%

The incidence of congenital hearing loss (> 50 dB) in Western Europe is approximately 1:1000 live births. In at least 50% of cases the cause is genetic and may be syndromic, autosomal recessive, or X-linked recessive. The most common inheritance pattern is autosomal recessive with many gene loci implicated. Even if the answer of autosomal recessive is given for both parts of this question the answer to c) is still > 95%, as the chance of both unrelated families having the same mutation is small and then only a 25% chance of passing both to the offspring.

5.3 Answer

a) **A** – Duodenal atresia

Note the 'double bubble' sign and absence of gas in the distal bowel.

5.4 Answer

a) **E** – Biliary colic
b) **A** – Abdominal ultrasound

Key points

■ Intermittent pain after mealtimes suggests biliary colic.

■ He is comfortable on examination and the pain is settling. The steady haemoglobin value excludes hepatic sequestration and Girdle syndrome.

Hepatic sequestration: occurs in all age groups, with abdominal distension, severe hypochondrial pain and rapidly enlarging liver.

Girdle syndrome: silent distended abdomen, commonly with hepatic enlargement and bilateral basal lung consolidation.

Gallstones are found in 30% of children and 70% of adults with sickle cell disease. Although generally asymptomatic, they may cause acute/chronic cholecystitis, biliary colic, or related acute pancreatitis. Some stones may be radiopaque so may be visible on plain abdominal X-ray. Ultrasound of the gall bladder is the most likely to confirm the diagnosis.

Acute cholecystitis is managed with analgesia, hydration and antibiotics. If recurrent problems occur, then elective laparoscopic (or occasionally open) cholecystectomy may be necessary, with careful preoperative preparation, often with exchange transfusion.

5.5 Answer

a) **1. C** – 3 years (a neat circle would be at 5 years)
    2. D – 4 years (shoe laces and buckles later)
    3. C – 3 years (will know surname by end of 3rd year)
    4. F – 6 years
    5. B – 2 years
    6. E – 5 years
    7. H – 8 years
    8. A – 1 year
    9. F – 6 years

There may be some leniency in the marking with milestones gained at an older age with some marks awarded for being 1 year out.

Reference

Griffiths, R, *The ability of young children: a comprehensive system of mental measurement for the first eight years of life.* The Test Agency Limited, 1984.

5.6 Answer

a) **B** – Erythema nodosum

Erythema nodosum (EN) is a nodular erythematous eruption generally confined to the anterior lower legs. The photo shows typical lesions which are redder than the bruises seen in the other conditions. A history of failure to thrive with a presentation of erythema nodosum should prompt investigations for inflammatory bowel disease.

5.7 Answer

a) A – Right-to-left shunting at the atrial level
    D – Critical pulmonary stenosis
    F – Patent ductus arteriosus with left-to-right shunting
b) D – Intravenous prostaglandin
c) D – Balloon valvular dilatation

A general approach and normal values for cardiac catheterisation are given in the answer to question 1.11. When each chamber is worked through sequentially as previously outlined, there is a fall in pressure between the right ventricle and pulmonary artery giving the diagnosis of pulmonary stenosis. There is a fall in the saturation at the left atrial level revealing right-to-left shunting through the foramen ovale. In critical pulmonary stenosis the infant is dependent on blood flow from left to right through a patent ductus arteriosus.

5.8 Answer

a) B – Short PR interval
    D – δ wave
b) C – Re-entry tachycardia

The ECG shown is of Wolff–Parkinson–White syndrome in which an accessory pathway (bundle of Kent) exists between the atria and the ventricles. This results in a shortened PR interval and a slurred upstroke to the QRS complex δ wave, best seen in V4 on this ECG. The most common arrhythmia is a re-entrant tachycardia; atrial fibrillation is a particular danger to these patients as it may progress to ventricular fibrillation.

5.9 Answer

a) D – Pityriasis versicolor

Pityriasis versicolor (tinea versicolor) is a fungal infection producing these patches of light colouration in skin. Pityriasis versicolor is caused by a yeast, *Malassezia furfur*, which is believed to be the parasitic form of a common saprophytic yeast *Pityrosporum orbiculare*, which may be found on normal skin. Although the infection is most common in tropical countries, it has a world-wide distribution. Climatic factors or exposure to sunlight are believed to trigger the infection in many cases.

Photo credit:

Dr P. Marazzi/Science Photo Library

5.10 Answer

a) **B** – Secondary cortisol deficiency
   C – Growth hormone deficiency
   G – Secondary hypothyroidism
b) **A** – Hydrocortisone
   D – Thyroxine
   G – Growth hormone

Growth hormone and cortisol responses to hypoglycaemia (ITT) are flat. In an ITT, if the hypoglycaemic response is adequate (decrease in blood sugar by 50% of starting value), then the GH should increase to > 13.5 mU/l and the cortisol level should increase by 100% of the basal value.

This is a hypothalamic response to TRH. Normally in response to TRH, the TSH levels should increase at 20 minutes and then decrease at 60 minutes, as should the prolactin level. In this case there is an exaggerated response to TRH with the TSH levels continuing to increase at 60 minutes.

Following cranial irradiation, GH insufficiency and secondary hypothyroidism are common. ACTH deficiency, gonadotrophin insufficiency and diabetes insipidus may occur but less commonly. Primary hypothyroidism and primary hypogonadism may also occur secondary to cranial irradiation.

5.11 Answer

a) **C** – Schwachmann–Diamond syndrome
b) **E** – Pancreatic enzyme supplements

Key points

- Neutropenia

- Faecal elastase deficiency indicates pancreatic enzyme deficiency

- Short stature

- Bony abnormalities

This syndrome of exocrine pancreatic hypoplasia, bone marrow abnormalities and metaphyseal dysplasia should be considered in the differential diagnosis of children with short stature and exocrine pancreatic failure in the presence of a normal sweat test. Pancreatic insufficiency may be diagnosed by measurement stool fat output (fat balance studies) and pancreatic stimulation tests. The latter test shows that after stimulation with cholecystokinin and secretin, pancreatic enzyme output is invariably low, but in cystic fibrosis, water and bicarbonate secretion is well preserved. Faecal elastase measurement is a simpler, non-invasive test of pancreatic function as this pancreatic enzyme is not digested or absorbed by the gut; therefore low levels indicate pancreatic exocrine insufficiency.

Sepsis is usually associated with neutropenia, which may be intermittent. Thrombocytopenia and hypoplastic anaemia are common.

5.12 Answer

a) **A** – *Candida* infection

In this case *Candida* is suggested because of the presence of satellite lesions visible on the abdomen.

Photo credit:

Dr P. Marazzi/Science Photo Library

5.13 Answer

a) **C** – Full septic screen including lumbar puncture and iv antibiotics
b) **E** – Congenital adrenal hypoplasia
c) **B** – Hydrocortisone
   D – Fludrocortisone
   E – Oral sodium supplements

This is a sick male infant who on admission has lost > 10% of his bodyweight and is passing dilute urine with inappropriately high sodium content. Obviously sepsis needs to be excluded and overwhelming urinary tract infection mimics this picture.

Congenital adrenal hyperplasia should be the working diagnosis once sepsis has been excluded. However, the results show that the

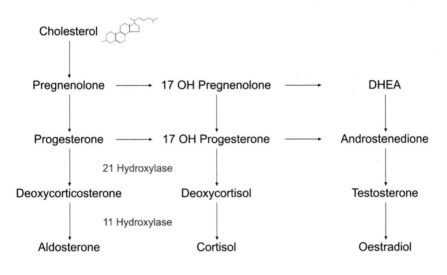

17-hydroxyprogesterone is low and distal metabolites are also low.

Congenital adrenal hypoplasia is less common than hyperplasia which itself is rare; 21-hydroxylase deficiency is the most common form of congenital adrenal hyperplasia.

5.14 Answer

a) **D** – CT brain scan
b) **A** – Sagittal sinus thrombosis

A clinical history of severe dehydration, but a full anterior fontanelle, suggests raised intracranial pressure. Normal fundi do not exclude this. Note the elevated CSF protein values (for normal range see answer to question 2.11).

The question is specific in asking for investigations to confirm a diagnosis, not an immediate investigation, so electrolytes would not be an appropriate answer.

Thrombosis of the cerebral veins occurs principally as a complication of severe dehydration, or as an extension of local infection. Sagittal sinus thrombosis occurs mainly in infants who are severely dehydrated, often as a consequence of diarrhoea, although one hopes with increasing understanding of oral rehydration therapy it will become less common. The venous obstruction leads to cerebral swelling with signs of raised intracranial pressure including stupor, coma and bulging fontanelle. Seizures and quadriparesis may occur, often with involvement of the extremities first.

Clinically, the condition may mimic encephalitis and metabolic encephalopathy. Practically, if there is a suspicion of raised intracranial pressure, a lumbar puncture should not be performed; normal fundi do not exclude intracranial pressure.

A CT scan may show the area of thrombosis, often with widespread haemorrhagic infarction of the brain. Cerebral angiography is of value in localising the site of obstruction. CSF examination is of little help: pressure is normally elevated, the fluid may be bloody and show white cells and an elevated protein content. In general the condition is managed supportively.

5.15 Answer

a) D – Hyphaema

This is a view of the eye of a patient suffering from hyphaema – bleeding into the anterior (front) chamber of the eye following an injury. Hyphaema often results from sports accidents, such as the impact of a cricket or squash ball. Vision becomes blurred while the blood and the aqueous humour (fluid inside the front chamber of the eye) are mixed, but it clears after the blood has settled (as here). The blood disappears within a few days.

Photo credit:

Dr Chris Hale//Science Photo Library

PERMISSIONS

PICTURE REFERENCE NUMBER: M155/425 (page 129)
TITLE: Hyphaema of the eye caused by a trauma
CREDIT: DR. CHRIS HALE/SCIENCE PHOTO LIBRARY

PICTURE REFERENCE NUMBER: M270/185 (page 50)
TITLE: Quinsy: peritonsillar abscess in the mouth
CREDIT: DR P. MARAZZI/SCIENCE PHOTO LIBRARY

PICTURE REFERENCE NUMBER: M220/101 (page 125)
TITLE: Candida nappy rash in a baby girl
CREDIT: DR P. MARAZZI/SCIENCE PHOTO LIBRARY

PICTURE REFERENCE NUMBER: M157/020 (page 79)
TITLE: Acute secretory otitis media
CREDIT: PROFESSOR TONY WRIGHT, INSTITUTE OF LARYN- GOLOGY &
OTOLOGY/SCIENCE PHOTO LIBRARY

PICTURE REFERENCE NUMBER: M160/012 (page 19)
TITLE: Fifth Disease: 'slapped cheek' marks on infant
CREDIT: DR H.C.ROBINSON / SCIENCE PHOTO LIBRARY

PICTURE REFERENCE NUMBER: M150/211 (page 103)
TITLE: Ectodermal dysplasia, EEC syndrome, feet
CREDIT: SCIENCE PHOTO LIBRARY

PICTURE REFERENCE NUMBER: M108/363 (page 55)
TITLE: LM of blood smear showing iron-deficiency anaemia
CREDIT: DR. E. WALKER/SCIENCE PHOTO LIBRARY

PICTURE REFERENCE NUMBER: M240/117 (page 122)
TITLE: Pityriasis versicolor: light patches on skin
CREDIT: DR P. MARAZZI/SCIENCE PHOTO LIBRARY

PICTURE REFERENCE NUMBER: M155/360 (page 75)
TITLE: Eyes of a child with congenital glaucoma
CREDIT: SUE FORD/SCIENCE PHOTO LIBRARY

PICTURE REFERENCE NUMBER: M240/226 (page 29)
TITLE: Squint caused by congenital cranial nerve palsy
CREDIT: DR P. MARAZZI/SCIENCE PHOTO LIBRARY

PICTURE REFERENCE NUMBER: M130/405 (page 71)
TITLE: Chickenpox lesion in the mouth of a child
CREDIT: DR P. MARAZZI/SCIENCE PHOTO LIBRARY

PICTURE REFERENCE NUMBER: M220/013 (page 95)
TITLE: Cafe au lait skin pigmentation
CREDIT: SCIENCE PHOTO LIBRARY

PICTURE REFERENCE NUMBER: M210/038 (page 90)
TITLE: Measles: Koplik's spots in mouth
CREDIT: DR P. MARAZZI/SCIENCE PHOTO LIBRARY

PICTURE REFERENCE NUMBER: M210/219 (page 90)
TITLE: Measles rash on a child's face
CREDIT: CNRI/SCIENCE PHOTO LIBRARY

PICTURE REFERENCE NUMBER: M200/089 (page 46)
TITLE: Erythema chronicum migrans rash from Lyme disease
CREDIT: JOHN RADCLIFFE HOSPITAL/SCIENCE PHOTO LIBRARY.

PICTURE REFERENCE NUMBER: M260/055 (page 40)
TITLE: Scarlet fever rash on a patient's tongue.
CREDIT: SCIENCE PHOTO LIBRARY

PICTURE REFERENCE NUMBER: M260/209 (page 40)
TITLE: Scarlet fever rash on a boy's upper body
CREDIT: BIOPHOTO ASSOCIATES/SCIENCE PHOTO LIBRARY

PICTURE REFERENCE NUMBER: M170/086 (page 82)
TITLE: Hypothyroidism: rash on an infant's body
CREDIT: BIOPHOTO ASSOCIATES/SCIENCE PHOTO LIBRARY

PICTURE REFERENCE NUMBER: M330/985 (page 58)
TITLE: Haematoma (bruise) on leg
CREDIT: ASTRID & HANNS-FRIEDER MICHLER/SCIENCE PHOTO LIBRARY

PICTURE REFERENCE NUMBER: M280/216 (page 5)
TITLE: Aphthous ulcer in a child's mouth
CREDIT: DR P. MARAZZI/SCIENCE PHOTO LIBRARY

INDEX

The page numbers in this index refer to the pages of the question and the answer. The word shown may not always be used in the question but may appear in the explanatory text of the answer

PasTest

PasTest has been established since 1972 and is the leading provider of exam-related medical revision courses and books in the UK. The company has a dedicated customer services team to ensure that doctors can easily get up to date information about our products and to ensure that their orders are dealt with efficiently. Our extensive experience means that we are always one step ahead when it comes to knowledge of the current trends and contents of the Royal College exams.

PasTest revision books have helped thousands of candidates prepare for their exams. These may be purchased through bookshops, over the telephone or online at our website. All books are reviewed prior to publication to ensure that they mirror the needs of candidates and therefore act as an invaluable aid to exam preparation.

100% Money Back Guarantee
We're sure you will find our study books invaluable, but in the unlikely event that you are not entirely happy, we will give you your money back – guaranteed.

Delivery to your Door
With a busy lifestyle, nobody enjoys walking to the shops for something that may or may not be in stock. Let us take the hassle and deliver direct to your door. We will despatch your book within 24 hours of receiving your order. We also offer free delivery on books for medical students to UK addresses.

How to Order
www.pastest.co.uk
To order books safely and securely online, shop at our website.

Telephone: +44 (0)1565 752000
Have your credit card to hand when you call.
Fax: +44 (0) 1565 650264
Fax your order with your debit or credit card details.

PasTest Ltd, FREEPOST, Knutsford, Cheshire WA16 7BR

Send your order with your cheque (made payable to PasTest Ltd) and debit or credit card details to the above address. (Please complete your address details on the reverse of the cheque.)

PasTest revision books for MRCPCH

MRCPCH 2 Paediatrics

SHORT CASES FOR THE PAEDIATRIC MEMBERSHIP
Mark Beattie, Andrew Clark, Anne Smith

1 901198 25 1

This book contains essential guidance for taking the Paediatric Clinical examination

- Systematic approach to Short Cases
- Useful schemes of Clinical examination
- Ideal for DCH candidates

£22.50

QUESTIONS FOR MRCPCH PART 2 WRITTEN EXAMINATION

Nick Barnes, Julian Forton 1 904627 16 1

- Contains 34 integrated questions with multiple photographs, radiological investigations and several stages of decision making
- Contains specialist, adolescent cases and additional cases covering commonly asked questions/essential knowledge
- Each integrated case-based question is accompanied by a comprehensive explanation and overview of the subject pertinent to the scenario

£34.50

To order, please contact PasTest on:
01565 752000

PasTest Ltd, FREEPOST, Knutsford, Cheshire, WA16 7BR
Fax: 01565 650264; E-mail: books@pastest.co.uk

Or order online at www.pastest.co.uk

PasTest Courses

PASTEST: the key to exam success, the key to your future

PasTest is dedicated to helping doctors to pass their professional examinations. We have 30 years of specialist experience in medical education and over 3000 doctors attend our revision courses each year.

Experienced lecturers:
Many of our lecturers are also examiners and teach in a lively and interesting way in order to:
- reflect current trends in exams
- give plenty of mock exam practice
- provide valuable advice on exam technique

Outstanding accelerated learning:
Our up-to-date and relevant course material includes MCQs, colour slides, X-rays, ECGs, EEGs, clinical cases, data interpretations, mock exams, vivas and extensive course notes which provide hundreds of high quality questions with detailed answers and explanations, succinct notes, diagrams and charts.

Personal attention:
Active participation is encouraged on these courses, so in order to give personal tuition and to answer individual questions our course numbers are limited.
Book early to avoid disappointment.

Choice of courses:
PasTest has developed a wide range of high quality interactive courses in different cities around the UK to suit your individual needs.

What other candidates have said about our courses:
'Absolutely brilliant – I would not have passed without it! Thank you.'
Dr Charitha Rajapakse, London.

Excellent, enjoyable, extremely hard work but worth every penny.'
Dr Helen Binns, Oxford.

For further details contact:
PasTest Ltd, Egerton Court, Parkgate Estate,
Knutsford, Cheshire WA16 8DX, UK.
Telephone: 01565 752000 Fax: 01565 650264
e-mail: courses@pastest.co.uk website: www.pastest.co.uk